D0562940

ENJOYING FOOD
ON A
DIABETIC DIET

ENJOYING FOOD

ON A

DIABETIC DIET

Edith M. Meyer

Dolphin Books
Doubleday & Company, Inc., Garden City, New York

Dolphin Edition: 1974. Originally published by
Doubleday & Company, Inc., in 1971.

ISBN: 0-385-01344-2
Copyright © 1971 by Edith M. Meyer
All Rights Reserved
Printed in the United States of America

To Dale

Foreword

The new diabetic is often distressed by his diagnosis. He is faced with the prospect of carrying out puzzling dietary regulations. Unless the disease is complicated or severe, his physician may not advise him to enter a hospital where he could be instructed properly, or even tell him to consult a dietician. The male victim has little interest in the details of the dietary prescription, which is difficult to carry out in his occupational situation, and may project this responsibility on to his wife. A printed form fails to meet the need, although usually some attempt is made to provide a list of standard foods to follow. It is necessary to learn how to vary the intake by substituting one food for another in the appropriate group. More sophisticated knowledge permits the patient to enjoy mixed dishes, even out at the restaurant or when entertaining guests, while still maintaining his diabetic program. This book to a large extent solves the problem.

Resolving to revise her food habits, the author, designated a new diabetic, sets out to organize a system. She dutifully records her food exchanges and loses her extra accumulation of sugar and weight. Badgering the manager, she calculates the food values of the various offerings on the supermarket shelves. She finally acquires an expertise which qualifies her to recommend concoctions even for the diabetic gourmet.

The early portion of the book entertains us with tales of her medical and laboratory experiences and provides practical hints, such as how to purchase bread and rolls, slice meat, and make gravy. The remainder consists of recipes presented in a practical and amusing manner, including the proper calculation of exchanges found in one serving. The meat and fish dishes are sensible, American, mouth-watering but healthful. Many instructions also apply to nondiabetics, especially if they are overweight, and can be employed for the whole family. Fruits, vegetables, and salads are dressed up for guests and children alike. Even the ubiquitous breakfast has its turn, and some menus offer special egg mixtures, dietetic pancakes or homemade jam.

Those mild diabetics who need to follow a reasonable program of sugar control with or without the addition of the oral antidiabetic agents will profit by following the author's suggestions. These recipes will *not* suit those diabetics who take insulin and wish to consult a precise reference for scientific calculation, which requires food exchange lists or quantitative weighed substitutions. Although several other diabetes cookbooks are available, not many offer such homespun, practical advice as is contained in this collection. If you have diabetes and have lost your zest for eating because of medical restrictions, relax. Try some of these ideas in your kitchen and enjoy mealtime again!

A. R. Colwell, Jr., M.D.

Preface

I like to eat. And I have eaten very well all my adult life—that is until I became diabetic. A small part of this book is about how I became ill and felt very hopeless and helpless and sorry for myself when I had to give up—I thought—my favorite pastimes, eating, cooking, and pleasing my guests.

You cannot all come to my house to eat what I cook now, and every bit of it from the Food Exchange List.[1] But you can eat with me, as what I eat is all here in this book, with every exchange and calorie calculated for you, your family, and your guests.

Gravy—fat free and better than what I used to make. And foolproof, too, never a lump.

Hash—I never thought I could have it again. So good my non-diet gourmet friends use my recipe.

Meats are not all boiled or broiled and they include minted lamb, gumbos, meat loaf, veal scallopine, chicken and artichokes—even macaroni and cheese.

Fruit jam—breakfast comes alive again.

I still like to eat. And I eat well and have almost

[1] See Appendix A.

forgotten that I am on a diet, and that all of my food is
from that once despised Food Exchange List.

Come to my house and good eating with these ways
to cook and eat.

Contents

DIARY ENTRY 1

The Diagnosis

First visit to the doctor, and exhausted after 14 hours' sleep. M.D. bouncing, cheerful: hate anyone with all that energy. Innumerable questions about ancestors and my bathroom frequency. Too tired to answer; shook head yes and no. "Glucose tolerance test." No meaning except that more had to happen before I could start to feel well. Another appointment made. Rules: no food, coffee O.K. Who cared; food didn't matter, coffee essential to get there. Whole thing seemed ridiculous. Can't get to work; can't think; all those people writing things down on clipboards. Felt like a bug specimen. "Now, just drink this." Cup of pale yellow liquid, tasted like essence of popsicle; pang of nausea. Many urine and blood samples. Medical technician utter bumbler at finding blood vessels; have seen dart throwers who made better hits. After hours of this, M.D., medical technician, nurse file in with pile of books for me, card for wallet, little plastic box. M.D. all cheery; why is he so happy? Seems delighted over his diagnostic skill. Wonder if I'm supposed to congratulate him. I don't. Expect Q & A period. Denied. Little box has metal medallion on little chain that I'm supposed to wear at all times; remembered old joke about fellow who got medal for V.D. Not funny anymore.

On the way home went to bakery and bought chocolate whipped cream pie for "last meal"; couldn't eat it. Too sick, so went to bed.

Read the books. Had to earn my Q & A period. Diabetes is the result of a disordered pancreas. Pancreas, who? I don't have any acquaintance with my pancreas. I am on very personal terms with my stomach, who has always been very cooperative in telling me what it likes and doesn't like. Heart has been a faithful friend, has gone properly to my throat with fear, has palpitated with young love, has thumped a warning on a mountain climb. In my head a brain who has helped me when I asked it to, and confused me when I let it have its own way. And now to be waylaid by my pancreas, which I don't know and which now dominates my life. On with the book. The pancreas produces insulin, which permits the body to metabolize sugars and starches and convert them into heat and energy. But mine doesn't do that anymore. I have to organize and maintain my own metabolism! I'm so disorganized I can't even get to work on time.

Read symptoms. Good grief, I'd had them all except real overweight. Fear increases. Really much sicker than old Ho Ho Ho had let on. Jumped to Index and found complications such as shock, coma, infected feet, bad eyes, skin pitting. No more reading out of that book.

I felt terrible and was scared and I have never had any faith in medical announcements such as "the patient is doing as well as could be expected." I've known for years that that meant anything short of calling in the family. I went into instant mourning for myself. My life as I knew it had ended. I had to tread a perilous tightrope consisting of measured work and rest interwoven with some kind of starvation diet.

Diet! Better read it. Book says bad eating habits correlate with disease. Thought of the baked potatoes yellow with butter to hold up the sour cream. Thought of my chocolate pie recipe with 12 ounces of chocolate bits under the whipped cream. I had seen myself as a gourmet—and horrors—what I really am is an addict, mainlining my way to coma—same thing.

Tried cheering myself up with the thought that I could "kick" it. If I couldn't kick it, I could commit suicide gloriously with two bottles of champagne and a platter of crepes Suzette. How elegant! Tried to decide whether to wear the pink pegnoir or the black silk opera suit.

Called friends to announce imminent death. Got nothing but stories of friend's friends who had been diabetics for years—ladies who had lived to eighty-seven, while delivering their home-grown vegetables to neighbors to the end, and one ego crusher even told me about somebody in her fifties who hikes with the Sierra Club to the top of Mount Whitney.

Friends no use. Doctor no use. All I have is a bottle of pills and a diet list.

I took a pill and that left me with the diet list. First column, glancing down it. All the raw vegetables I wanted. Okra? Poke? Rhubarb without sugar.

Try next column. Bread, bisquit, roll: one!

Next was meat—love meat. This will save me. "3 in. ×2 in. by ⅛ in." Four bites! I really had been sentenced; prisoners would rattle their dishes, throw their silverware, and maybe even set the dining room on fire.

Read it all, almost all. Over 20 years of cooking knowledge blanked out. I was worse than condemned.

Back to bed. Catnaps with much poor thinking. Resolved. I am a food addict. What do addicts do—cold turkey! I'll go on the diet and never swerve.

Didn't swerve until the middle of the first breakfast, and also didn't notice list 7, *Foods That Need Not Be Measured.*

DIARY ENTRY 2

Cold Turkey

Resolved: Kick my food habits.

FIRST DAY. On 1300 calories a day. Have to lose 7 pounds. Seems simple.

Up at six; half an hour early to eat breakfast. Haven't eaten breakfast for 20 years. Book says metabolic balance important. Must eat breakfast or freak-out.

Got out egg, 1 slice bread, orange juice, milk, measured 1 teaspoon of butter. Drank O.J. Nice. Put half of butter in small pan and tried to scramble egg. Egg stuck in pan. Made toast. The ½ teaspoon of butter left covered upper quarter of toast. Ate bites of egg I could get out of pan, and the toast at the buttered end. Ate bite of toast without butter. Ugh! Tried to wash down toast with milk; hate milk. Threw out rest of egg, toast, milk. Left dirty pan—no time left.

Went to work. Took diet.

No cafeteria at our office. Only restaurant is Italian. A catering truck comes by four times a day. Look at sandwiches: each made with about ⅛ inch of meat. Need two of these for meat exchange. Bought two at 45¢ each. Threw away 3 breads to make new sandwich as I had only 1 bread exchange. Bought milk, 20¢, orange, 20¢, banana, 20¢. Lunch $1.50. Real food available at Italian restaurant for $1.25. Didn't drink milk. Threw away one-half of banana as required. Wasn't hungry anyway.

Still terribly thirsty and weak. Tried a diet drink. Tasted terrible. Threw away. Took nap in ladies' room. Drank coffee. Went home 2 hours early.

Shopped for dinner, diet in hand.

For dinner, 1 cup of spinach, no butter. Just salt. Horrible. Might as well cook weeds. Broiled one-half a chicken. Cut two slices as directed. Not enough. One-half cup rice. One bread. Spread butter on one half bread, folded bread, couldn't taste the butter. Didn't make it on the milk again. Ate peach. Went to bed, very unhappy.

SECOND DAY. Couldn't get to work. Decided to try diet as I had read on a "Sample Meal Plan." Shopped before breakfast for all in plan. Got dizzy.

Breakfast. O.J. again. Still O.K. Took ¾ cup cereal flakes, added 2 tablespoons light cream. Cream didn't cover. Kept stirring to cover and added milk. Fiddled around with it so long it got mushy. Left with egg to eat and had already used bread exchange. Can't eat a naked egg. Hard-boiled it for snack.

Snack. Egg still seemed naked, even dipped in salt. Ate half.

Lunch. Got out 3 sardines and proper amount of cheese. Tried to make sandwich out of this on one piece of bread. All kept falling out. Made salad. Measured 1 tablespoon French dressing. Tossed salad. Every sixth or seventh bite had some dressing. Not a salad. Sandwich terrible. Ate half, put rest on sideboard. Ate pear and peach. Very nice. Daughter came home. Nosy as usual. Sees sardine and cheese sandwich on sideboard. "Mom! You made lunch for Algernine" (her pet rat). "That's my lunch," I muttered. She didn't believe it. Fed to rat. Algernine berserk with joy. Ye gods, this lunch is rat food.

Dinner. Still following "Sample" meal even though lunch flunked. Made beef broth out of bouillon cube. Awful. Beef broth is what you start with to make onion soup with cheese in it. Why do I have to eat ingredients instead of food? Ate roast beef, plain vegetables, 2 rolls. Used all butter on one. Ate other without butter. Beats dry toast. Ate watermelon, fine. "Sample" called for 6 small nuts. Why on earth would anyone eat 6 nuts? Everyone knows about 1 peanut.

Every day for 3 weeks I followed the diet, right off the exchange list, to the exact exchange. Results:

Grocery bill tripled (throwaways)
Lost 14 pounds, not 7 (throwaways)
Weak as the famous cat—but diabetic symptoms except for weakness were gone.

A new nitty-gritty problem. Judge and jury were right. Pills and diet have worked. But *I can't stand the food.* I'll waste away. Malnutrition will overcome me. I'll look like a yogi.

DIARY ENTRY 3

Pavlov's Dog

I went back to the doctor to explain slow starvation. Sent to closed door office, *the* office, the one with the books. An overwhelming smell of sweet chocolate. I asked him, "What are you doing in here, making fudge?" Says no, asks why. I explain and he remembers a friend in on lunch hour who had eaten a candy bar 1 hour and 15 minutes before. He was delighted as he said he knew I had not eaten any chocolate as my sense of smell had a dropped threshold like that. Dropped threshold! I tried to continue the conversation, no time for him.

I explained the reason for the visit, and got the third degree. Finally I admitted all. Well, not *all*. I did admit that I didn't like the milk and didn't drink it. After all it's a sin not to like milk; ask any mother, regardless of race, or religion. Churches and schools have milk funds, even the United Nations.

M.D. utterly exasperated, as I had expected. But not about the milk, just about not eating my proper amounts of food. I got two "go's." Up to 1500 calories. And he explained that many diet experts do not feel that non-childbearing adults need very much milk. He allowed me to convert my milk exchanges to meat exchanges,[1] and dismissed the case for the afternoon, before I even got to the vegetables.

Rushed to the car, and got out the diet; 1300 column out, 1500 column in—2 meat exchanges were elevated to three for dinner. I did an instant calorie conversion in my head, and rushed to the nearest market and bought real filets mignons for dinner. I charcoal broiled them, and ate a whole real steak. Never had I eaten anything like it. No food had ever tasted close to it. It was the filet of filets.

Funny about that steak. I never had gotten a good steak from that market before.

"Dropped threshold." My thinking was coming back, and I remembered dimly that old psychology course where we learned that threshold is the lowest point of sensitivity, including taste, smell, pain, and all. I can taste better? Ridiculous. Was it? Curiosity prevailed.

(My parents would never answer a question. If you want to know something, "Look it up." Consequently, I never remember much, but I really know how to look it up.)

Out of the steak reverie and to the library. On the way I thought of Pavlov and his dog. Dr. Pavlov rang a bell and his dog had been trained to salivate. He didn't salivate to pepper, doughnuts, apple pie, or fudge. Just a stupid bell. There is more to this; I'll look it up.

I brought back a load of books with heady titles. Thresholds, there were a whole universe of thresholds, but briefly, here is the taste and smell nutshell.

First lecture: Your tongue is limited—it can only taste

---

[1] The proper exchange for 1 milk exchange is 1 scant bread exchange, 1 meat exchange, and 1 fat exchange.

salt, sweet, sour, and bitter. Your sense of smell is capable of hundreds of subtle differences, and these combine with the taste buds in the tongue for your whole food sensitivity. If you don't believe this, hold your nose the next time you are eating (at home). It is only because of smell that we have really flavorsome food, gourmets, and good cooks.

Second lecture: If any heavy salt, sweet, etc., solution is run over your tongue, in 2 minutes you can no longer taste it. And with an average odor, in 3 minutes, you can't smell it. This is called adaptation; in case you are a looker-upper, it will save you a trip.

Where if that was all, did the rest of my food-tasting habits come from? Back to the books; all the rest are just plain old habit, like Pavlov's dog, or dropping the left shoe before the right.

I remembered my childhood eating. The great depression was on, and my family fully participated—not on purpose. Also my mother really didn't cook very well (I'll tell you that in the Vegetable chapter) except for lemon pie and orange marmalade. We hunted for part of our food, and got mostly jack rabbits—that's what there were most of. Well, if I learned to like jack rabbit (you have to spit out the buckshot, too) I could learn to eat anything. All of the rich food tastes I have were gotten after I was twenty-one. And the steak really did taste better, because of all of the very plain food I had eaten, which had lowered my taste threshold.

Now, where did I stand? I had lost my symptoms and weight, had "dropped my threshold," which meant I was ready for new taste experiences, had "adapted out" some old tastes, but I still couldn't stand the non-salad salads, boiled meat, dry toast, and boiled vegetables.

DIET ENTRY 4

A Hard Look at the Diet—
OR WHY I HAD TO CHANGE SUPERMARKETS

I began to develop the exchanges given with each of the recipes in this book, and they are not random guesses. They began as measurements gleaned from a research mission that took me deep into hostile territory. I ferreted out information by working under the very noses of the authorities in my neighborhood supermarket, and when the true nature of my activities became known, I was immediately declared persona non grata and I now do my shopping several blocks further down the street.

But I came away with my precious calculations. I broke the code! I had started to escape from boiled food and all by calculation:

". . . The first step in the computation is to figure out the largest constituent, the carbohydrate," says one nutritionist in his explanation of the food exchange system. I read on with interest, clutching my slide rule. The equation went on:

$$8.2\% \text{ of } 227 \text{ gm.}-X \text{ gm. CHO} \qquad 227$$
$$0.082 \times 227 - 18.6 \text{ gm. CHO} \qquad \times.82$$

$$\underline{454}$$
$$1816$$
$$\overline{18.614}$$

By this method one can determine that a can of fruit cocktail contains 2 fruit exchanges.

"Hmn," I thought, and carefully laid the paper down and put the slide rule on it. I would obviously have to restock the kitchen with a ruler to measure the meat, a tape measure for fruits (cantaloupe, ¼, 6 inch dia.), and a scale that weighed in grams—but what was I doing! I had already been told I could use the Food Exchange List.

Back to the list: Resolved to really understand it.

"Cherries," it said, "10 large."

"Large as compared to what?" My scientific mind rebelled. There are cherries and then there are cherries. How large is a large fig? Grapes, 12 . . . what kind?

I remembered more of my psychology courses. Mature people are supposed to have a "tolerance for ambiguity" it said somewhere. But I was not about to measure meat to ⅛ inch on the one hand and rest on my tolerance for ambiguity when it came to shrimp. Besides, I knew full well that if I let ambiguity into my diet, it would soon take over completely, and I'd be right back to the champagne and chocolate candy in no time at all.

The library failed me. The Department of Agriculture Handbook talks in pounds or grams, and I wanted volume, and the Encyclopedia Britannica predictably treated shrimp as a zoological entity, and not something you eat, and I still didn't know what 12 grapes were.

I was on my way home when the solution hit me, and I whipped into the supermarket parking lot—a giant research library! I *grabbed* my notebooks and pencils and ran to the seafood counter; I was still intrigued with the shrimp problem. I rang the bell and the butcher appeared.

"Would you please weigh five of the small shrimp?" I requested sweetly.

"Now, would you please weigh five of the medium shrimp." And so we progressed through all the available sizes. He weighed and I jotted it all down carefully.

"Thank you ever so," I murmured, departing without purchasing anything, leaving the bewildered butcher surrounded by piles of shrimp.

I counted veal chops per pound, lamb chops, all the way down the counter, aware of the butcher's gaze following me, and when I left 2 hours later (I had to go home and fix dinner) I knew what I had suspected was true. What the diet or any good cookbook calls medium shrimp, the supermarket calls large. Really large shrimp are called "giant" or "super" or prawns, even if they aren't. But now I was on the way to establishing a common language between the dieter and the advertisers.

The next day I went back to the supermarket armed with a list of questions.

"Phony sour creams," I prodded. "What oil do they use?"

"How much fat is there in a bouillon cube?"

"If sugar isn't listed, isn't there really any sugar in the canned tomatoes?"

"How much fat is in the bologna?"

The poor dear really tried, but he didn't know; as an aside the FDA doesn't either, in all cases. And I went to the bread row, directly in view of the suspicious manager.

I counted the slices of bread in large, medium, and small sizes. I did the English muffins, brown-and-serve rolls, and wrote down all the numbers of slices in pounds and ounces, as the manager became more agitated. A clerk appeared with more bread and started restocking and straightening up all the shelves, while I went on to the vegetable and fruit departments.

I spent an hour on grapes. I counted grapes in bunches—Thompson seedless, Malaga, Tokay—I weighed and counted and there it was! The answer to one of my questions: 40 Thompson seedless grapes equal 1 fruit exchange.

I weighed all kinds of oranges, one at a time. The manager was still watching, and the vegetable man was madly cleaning out old lettuce, and I spent the rest of the day on fruits and vegetables.

Ensuing days were spent on canned goods, and powdered and canned milk, and I made a thorough sweep of the delicatessen, scribbling the prices of packaged meat per pound, and other valuable bits of information.

When I finally had enough information, I approached the manager. He was on full alert by now, and almost saluted when I addressed him.

I patiently explained that the hamburger was almost white with fat and that I thought he really should speak to the butcher about it.

"I don't understand," he muttered, in what surely must have been a gross understatement.

"Well," I said, "suppose you are a diabetic like me and you have to calculate all the food you eat, and . . ."

"You mean you're not from the Bureau of Standards." His words were like little pellets of ice.

"Oh, no, I'm just trying to improve my diet."

Every now and then I go back to that market. The manager always hides when he sees me coming, and in retrospect I think he shows amazing self-control. The vegetable people disappear, and the butcher denies having any other pork, beef, etc., except what's out.

I console myself with the thought that all of us pioneers seem to stir up muddy water. It's a good thing I never wanted to be a missionary. I would have probably been cooked by order of the tribe's public relations man.

But I don't have to defer to that tolerance for ambiguity now, and I can cook in plain English, the sardine sandwich days are over and the food list is what it is intended to be—a list and not a cookbook.

HOW TO EAT—BE SELFISH

Introduction to New Eating Patterns

During all of this turmoil I read this discouraging word:

"My soul is dark with stormy riot,
Directly traceable to diet."
                                    Samuel Hoffenstein

My soul had improved no end after the apple or 40 grapes had hit me on the head and I had finally realized that the American Diabetic Association's food list wasn't a cookbook. That was the real beginning of the recipes in this book, but there are more to recipes than meet the tummy; that, of course, is our problem in the first place. I had received many wonderful brochures from the American Diabetic Association and their information is included in many of the recipes but there is more to eating enjoyably on a diabetic diet than just having some good recipes.[1]

My soul was still troubled by how I was going to discipline myself forever and still follow my food rules. I mulled at length and while mulling I was interrupted by my junior high daughter,

"Can you give me three reasons for the fall of the Roman Empire?"

[1] The American Diabetic Association also has an official cookbook. Check with your local chapter to obtain one.

"Sugar, fat, and calories," I replied.

"Huh?"

Fat! Where had I read it? I got out all my stacks of paper, found what I had read by many diet authorities but not grasped as a way to have a non-diet dinner.

> There is a wonderful-for-us peculiarity of fat digestion. All of the exchanges must be eaten at the meal and in the amount allowed *except* for fats. Fat exchanges may be saved up during a day, but not for more than one day, and used in another meal!

This means that perhaps on a day when you would like a salad with more than 2 teaspoons of mayonnaise—just not enough to make a salad taste good—you can save fat exchanges for that extra good salad. Or you can save a couple of fat exchanges and have artificially sweetened *real* whipped cream on strawberries. This, on a 1500-calorie-a-day diet, means that 4 fat exchanges, which are allowed, plus 2 fat exchanges saved from fat-free milk, equals 6 fats for dinner. And, of course, you should eat the exact amount of fat you are supposed to eat every day. You wouldn't want to do this every day as you want to maintain a balance of all of your different foods, and also if you saved fat exchanges every day it would become as tedious as eating right off the food list. But if you can save a fat exchange by eating Fat-Free Gravy, you have one to use for buttered peas.

Real dinner! Cooking for everyone in the family instead of goodies for everyone else and doleful little separate dishes for you and me. Going out to dinner without making everyone squirm when the butter goes by. Real salad. Vichyssoise. Sauce-sauce. Potatoes au gratin!

I had a new project: save fat all day. First, I didn't
see how I could eat dry toast for breakfast. Simple answer.
I can't and probably you can't either. A mass-produced
grocery store bread without something on it is unedible.
Diabetics have an increased appetite for bread and other
starches and the staff of life is full of twigs—French
bread, rolls, special bakery breads, brown-and-serve rolls,
English muffins, Melba toast—glorious arrays. Heat them
up, a good hot roll doesn't need butter. Buy half a dozen
of the best-looking ones you can find—hide them from
the rest of the family and start eating them for breakfast.
Just don't start with "diet" bread, it tastes like ground
cardboard.

For lunch, buy good bakery bread for sandwiches. Soft
little rolls such as little sesame seed or potato rolls are
great for sandwiches, too. Also, there are many good frozen
raw breads available. These are as much like homemade
bread as you can buy, and they are not expensive. You
can also make them into rolls, for your butterless breakfast
rolls or for dinner rolls. At today's prices you cannot really
save money, or energy, by making your own bread.

If you work or your husband is the patient, taking your
lunch to work helps to control your food. Beginning with
the good bakery bread, if you can't eat a ham, tomato,
and lettuce sandwich without butter or mayonnaise, with
the ham recommended in the meat section, you don't de-
serve good ham. Or leftover sirloin roast, with salt and
pepper, and maybe thinly sliced dill pickles in it? By the
way, part of the trick of eating butterless sandwiches is in
the slicing of the meat. Have a knife so sharp the police
would confiscate it, and slice your 1 or 2 meat exchanges

so thin you can almost see through them. This changes the whole sandwich taste.

When my doctor gave me permission to substitute part of my milk exchange for meat exchanges the first thing I did was to go up to two sandwiches. The way you can do this and stay within your bread allowance is to have the bakery slice your bread at half thickness so that two slices of bread equals 1 bread exchange. Two sandwiches are better than one, even if it only looks better. And if your husband is the patient, this will be a real morale lifter. That one little sandwich looks pretty sad to a guy who is used to eating.

So I became selfish. Everyone has been picking on "Mom" for years: sociologists, psychologists, "pop" writers, women's magazines. Fine. Give them something to pick on. Your special foods cost a little more. Hoard your goodies, and don't bother with an outdated conscience. You aren't depriving your greedy little sticky-fingered children, who are going to try to look like CARE advertisements because Mommy is eating something they don't have. They would rather have hamburgers on buns they understand, instead of little rolls with funny seeds on them. Let them eat cake—you can't. Save the leftover sirloin, ham, and turkey for yourself. Look at what the kids get, a happy, healthy mother instead of a sick grouch.

Before you start cooking, a couple of directions are needed. Any fats you save from fat-free milk must be saved from the milk you drink. The recipes use whole milk, as fat-free milks do not always work well, in fact, they will "do in" many recipes.

All of the recipes in this book are based on a 1500-

calorie-a-day diet. Most of them are very easy to increase or decrease.

"How to Eat" continues throughout the book. When I learned how to eat, I escaped from what I thought was a trap.

DIARY ENTRY 5

Rediscovering the Wheel

MONDAY Spent a few days munching 40 grapes, many 5 shrimp, much chicken. Stewed some of the chicken. Rotisseried others. Haven't ever left depression days so save string, leftovers such as the chicken parts and juices.

TUESDAY Just stood at dinnertime, staring at plain raw rice. Not again. Leftover chicken juice. Uhm. Used the chicken broth instead of water, little MSG (monosodium glutamate), seasoning salt, rice. Got super rice and no butter needed. Jewish penicillin, no. Jewish nectar, yes.

Called my gourmet friend Alberta in rapture. Alberta not raptured. Says how could I forget I always knew that.

Hung up and contemplated navel. Concluded I'd been like the first-year medical student who thought he had every disease in the book, but no cure.

Spent 2 hours finding old recipes. Have mathematical friend who has calculated the average women spends 2 months a year just looking for things. Have gone above average.

MONDAY What a triumph! Had friends for dinner on Sat. Used refound recipe for an astounding standing rib roast. Got shrewd, as was still drunk with power since chicken broth. Removed roast from pan. Rushed pan to freezer. Gave guests another drink. Chipped fat from cold pan. Measured and made gravy using arrowroot with the shimmering brown juice in the pan, and got Fat-Free Gravy! Delectable, a creation. Had idle daydream on receiving a Nobel prize for cooking as Fat-Free Gravy was obviously a medical break-through. Heart and diabetic patients throwing flowers. Must call Alberta and report lifesaving creation. She said, "Oh, you mean as the French do it, *au jus?*" I had rediscovered the wheel.

Giving up the Nobel prize was easy to take. At least I no longer had to figure out how to spread 1 teaspoon of butter over a serving of mashed potatoes. And I had a fat exchange left over.

THURSDAY Got a little lazy and tried commercial broths and bouillon cubes. Couldn't tell how much fat was in the cubes, and the canned broths are flat-tasting and not strong enough for the gravy.

MONDAY Spent 3 frenzied days making stocks and bouillons and freezing them. Spent 2 more frenzied days driving around giving them away when the freezer fan broke.

Learned a lot though. They cost pennies. Will also tolerate the sloppiest cooking. Practically no rules and almost anything will work.

HOW TO EAT

Stocks, Bouillons, and Fat-Free Gravy or HOW TO MAKE A SILK PURSE OUT OF A SOW'S EAR

The stocks and bouillons in this cookbook are the means to eating high on the hog and to balancing the pleasure of elegant foods with savings in the fat exchanges and savings in the purse.

Several kinds of bouillons and stocks are needed for many reasons. First, they are free on our diet, so that they can become the basis of many foods and with different methods of seasoning you can have different flavors. They can become soup, turn into goulash, be part of an oriental dinner, start sauces, and, most marvelously, can turn into fat-free gourmet gravy which you may—diabetics, heart patients, chubbies—all eat. And the chicken bouillon is what raises vegetables out of the doldrums of plain boiled hospital-flavored lumps into individual succulent bites.

There is only one constant rule on how to prepare stocks and bouillons, thick or thin. All of them must be prepared the day before (or weeks before, as they freeze beautifully) they are eaten. The reason for this is of utmost importance —to get rid of that "low on the hog" fat. This is done by chilling the whole potful overnight, and then lifting off every last chip of fat that has risen to the top. In other recipe books there is usually some direction to "skim off the fat" during the preparation period. Don't even try. You can't get all the fat out when it is warm.

The best part of our sow's ear is that the most delicious stocks are made from leftovers. Beef rib bones, steak bones, chicken parts, almost any meats, and all beef "drippings."

For instance, the recipe for Astounding Standing Rib Roast will make you feel when you taste it that you should be cooking for kings. But, when you serve it, don't serve the rib bones, just cut closely up to them. After all, most people don't pick them up for that "close to the bone flavor" no matter how much they want to. If you are eating in a restaurant, ask for your ribs in a "doggy bag" and ask for everyone else's in your party too. Or ask for steak bones, and anything else you can get out of the restaurant and still be legal.

BEEF STOCK

(*From leftovers and for gravy*)

Cut the leftover beef rib bones apart and add steak bones, leftover scraps of beef, anything beefy. Put them in a large pot. Cover with water, about an inch over the tops of the bones. Add a teaspoon of seasoning salt, a teaspoon of MSG, a few celery leaves, a couple slices of onion. Wait until it is cooked to salt it, as the meat was probably already salted during the original cooking. Cover and simmer 4 to 5 hours. Chill in the pot overnight. Chip off fat. The stock should be a rich brown, and slightly jellied. Warm it up, remove the bones, feed the meat to the cat, and strain the liquid. Store in containers of 1 cup each. I would suggest freezing it, since this thick stock will spoil quite easily.

Maybe you feel this is a lot of work. It really isn't unless you cook it 1 cup at a time. Save up, and keep frozen, the scraps and bones until you can make a really large amount. Then you have only one big greasy pot day. But let's get to the gravy.

FAT-FREE GRAVY

Get out a cupful of the frozen Beef Stock. Put it in a saucepan on low heat, and it will thaw very quickly. This gravy is easier to make than "forbidden" gravy. The secret, besides the fatlessness, is arrowroot. You only use one-half of the amount of arrowroot for thickening as you would flour or cornstarch, and it is much more digestible. Remember the arrowroot cookies that babies eat? And arrowroot mixes more quickly and without lumps. (You can also make this gravy from fresh drippings if you have enough. Put your roast aside, quickly put the pan in the freezer, and chip the fat off. Measure your liquid and add water to make even cupfuls.)

1 cup Beef Stock
1 tablespoon arrowroot

Put a couple of tablespoons of stock in a cup and mix the arrowroot with it. Heat the stock to a simmer, pour in the arrowroot mixture, and stir until it thickens. You have now obtained freedom from dry potatoes and noodles.

1 cupful of gravy equals ½ bread exchange   34 calories
¼ cup (for one) has 8 bread exchange calories!

(Do not freeze at this point, it will separate. Just make enough for one meal.)

BEEF STOCK

(*From scratch*)

If you have no leftover bones and want to make gravy or other things such as Dirty Eggs (see Index), here is how you start from the beginning.

3 pounds raw beef ribs, cut up, or soup bones that are meaty.

Shake up with 2 teaspoons of flour and 2 teaspoons of salt.

Preheat the oven to 450° F. Put ribs in a flat pan and cook until they are very dark brown. Now, you proceed just exactly as in the Beef Stock recipe just given, seasonings, water, cooking, and all. You will probably get about 2 cups of strained stock.

As you can see, this is a little more work than just saving leftovers, so try to save them and spare yourself the extra steps. Also, depending on the meat, the stock might turn out a little pale. If you are cooking for yourself and don't care, well, no problem. But if you are cooking it for people (husbands) who expect gravy to be brown, for heaven's sake, color it with brown food coloring. Everyone in the commercial world does it, you aren't being dishonest. If you can't find it, go to a bakery where they do special decorating and ask the decorator to get you some when he orders. Explain why, and when he realizes how little you need, he'll probably sell you some, or just give it to you.

CHICKEN STOCK AND CHICKEN
FAT-FREE GRAVY

Chicken gravy stock and chicken gravy are made exactly the way the Beef Stock is. Save all those brown necks, wing ends, backs, and leftovers, including drippings and crumbs. Use the same recipe as for Beef Stock—same seasonings except add a bay leaf. Do all of the chilling, defatting, and freezing. Then you make the chicken gravy exactly as the beef gravy. If this gravy is pale, add a few drops of yellow food coloring. These are available in those little cake coloring kits; almost all markets have them.

BOUILLONS

Use your best cooked leftovers for the gravies and stocks; bouillons are just simple soups, and you can use cheap raw cuts of meat. Just cook these until they taste good, meaty and flavorful, chickeny or beefy, as the case may be. Make a lot of chicken bouillon to freeze, as many recipes in this book call for it.

CHICKEN OR BEEF BOUILLON

2 pounds raw tails, wings, or backs of chicken
OR
2 pounds beef soup bones
1 tablespoon salt
1 teaspoon MSG
1 bay leaf for chicken OR
¼ teaspoon marjoram for beef
Celery leaves
2 quarts water

Put all of it into a pot and simmer until flavorsome, about 3 hours. Cool overnight. Remove fat, warm, strain, and freeze in little containers in 1-cup amounts. This shouldn't take more than 5 minutes to put together.

It is not difficult to understand why we do all of this for both the thick stocks and the thin bouillons instead of using canned broths or bouillon cubes. For one thing, both cubes and canned broths contain fat and you can't tell how much. Second, neither is strong enough to make the gravy. Next, this, though more work, is cheaper. But remember, the more you make at once, the easier it is. And last, both your own stock and the bouillons will taste incredibly better.

HOW TO EAT

Meat

Meat is where I live. I didn't have any trouble adjusting to the meat part of the diet, except I now had an excuse to buy what I liked best.

You have the same diet I do, so it's where you live, too. If you used to dip everything in batter and deep fry it (delicious), that's out, unless you are very, very clever at calculating the fat exchanges used. And if you change to plain boiling, the meat is simply ready for a "decent" burial—even the most sadistic dietician wouldn't do a thing like that.

Meat is the best part of any diet. Go to the store after you read this, look at all the meat to get an educated eye—pick a recipe and go! All of the recipes in the book are for the whole family. If you have large eaters, double the recipes and eat one-eighth instead of the one-fourth usually called for.

Look at your diet and figure out how much milk you can trade for meat.[1] For me, that changed a 2-ounce filet mignon to a 4-ounce filet mignon and I don't have to explain what that means. But be sure to leave the exact exchange substitute to your doctor.

[1] See Footnote, page 9.

Except for a few rules and a little information, you don't have to become a meat expert; you just have to be stubborn. Don't let the butcher tell you what "good" meat is; a lot of them don't know and they are in the position of having to sell what they have in stock. The best thing to do is to trade with a privately owned butcher shop. These people usually know more about meat and are dedicated to the fussy eater. Tell him your problem, and when he discovers that you are going to buy more than fat-free ground round, and buy *all* of the time, he's yours.

If you have a good supermarket, just follow the advice below. (In a supermarket watch out for those pink lights in the meat case. When you move a package of ground meat a few steps away from the counter, a lot of that pretty pink meat turns out to be lots of nice white fat.) If you are for one reason or other stuck with a supermarket, and the meat does not meet our standards, don't argue with the butcher, he just works there. Send a polite letter to the management, explain the problem, and tactfully point out that there are 5 million heart patients, 5 more million diabetics, and 10 or 20 million overweight customers, and that the market is not getting its share of the business. This will be very well understood.

For fish, just as with butcher shops, try to find a privately owned fish store. Fresh fish looks fresh. It kind of gleams, and stands up firmly rather than being softly draped over another.

The kinds of meat available to heart patients and diabetics are a little different from each other, but for the heart patient the difference is the emphasis on low cholesterol and/or fat. The diabetic is allowed a little more variety, but some of the heart rules are so good that the diabetic should adopt them. Beside the fats we should not overeat, there are good economic reasons for avoiding certain meats. Here is one good example. (Heart patients, look at the diabetic Food Exchange List, Appendix A, at the back of the book to follow this.) Thinking of sandwiches (remember the chapter on how to eat), let's compare bologna and leftover rump roast.

One pound of boneless rump cooked medium yields 12 meat exchanges and as of today costs $1.35 a pound.

One pound of bologna yields 9 meat exchanges and 3 fat exchanges (cut as Food Exchange List) and costs 90 cents a pound.

I reduced the beef by 25 per cent for shrinkage and fat trimming and then calculated the cost per meat exchange each. At today's prices, both worked out to 15 cents per meat exchange, and with no loss of precious fat exchanges for the beef!

Aside from the beautiful reality that roast beef doesn't cost more than bologna, that illustration is included so you will be prepared for what may come to you as a shock. When you read the meat list given next, you are going to have a moment of panic or despair. Please don't scream, "I can't afford it!" You can't not afford it. First, you can't eat all that fat, and second, your children should not be raised on fatty meat. Third, these better cuts of meat do not need to be cooked well done: medium or rare, depending on the cut of the meat, tastes better and the difference in shrinkage can go as high as 35 per cent. A sirloin roast cooked rare shrinks only about 5 per cent.

Fourth, you can eat ample amounts of chicken or turkey, neither of which are expensive, and many fish are inexpensive too. (Although, some hobby fishermen's wives have privately told me that the "free" fish costs about $20 a pound.)

MEATS TO USE:

Chicken, turkey, squab—lean, and don't eat the skin (too bad)

Fish—fresh or frozen, smoked, canned (except in oil)[2]

Veal—any lean cut

Beef, ground—round or chuck, fat trimmed first

Roasts—lean rump, lean chuck, round, O-bone, sirloin tip

Steaks—lean flank, sirloin, round, club, T-bone, filet

Lamb—lean leg, loin, shoulder

Pork—lean loin, ham

Ham—center cuts, butt, picnic, Canadian bacon

I avoid duck, goose, spareribs, short ribs, fatty roasts, mutton, fatty frankfurters, fatty sausage and lunch meats, and fatty hamburger for two reasons. One, unless you can buy the very best or you know the fat content, many of these meats on the market today exceed the fat already calculated for you in your meat exchange. And, two, I don't want to pay for chunks of fat, visible or invisible.

That's all you have to remember, and it's sort of what you really knew in your heart anyway. The rest you can do with a trained eye.

Just learn new meat traffic signals: red means go, white means stop. In beef or pork look for large expanses of red or pink (pork) meat. Little runs or threads of fats (considered gourmet, but not by you) are out. Those gourmet cuts are "Prime" and are the really expensive meats—we at least don't have to pay those prices. And

[2] See fish chapter for "free" fats in fish.

at the other end of the price range, if you pay 65 cents for cheaper, fattier cuts and throw away the fat, you are paying $1.00 a pound anyway. Large, whole pieces of fat that can be cut out are just not a good buy, unless it is a sale to end all sales. If it is, you could buy, say, an oven pot roast, cut out the fat before cooking, and either tie it or skewer it back together. That keeps the meat moist and the shrinkage down. When you buy the better cuts, look at both sides of the meat. With a roast that you are going to cook either uncovered in the oven or barbecue (true roasting) about a quarter inch of fat should be left on, again for shrinkage and moisture. You don't eat it, just like the turkey skin.

With poultry, make the effort to find truly fresh poultry. I mean "straight from the farm" and not frozen before you see it. This has no dietary importance, but if you live in a big city, you probably don't even remember what fresh chicken or turkey tastes like. Well, it's just like a different food, with a succulence and chickenness that will bring tears of childhood memories to your eyes.

As for ham, almost every large meat producer makes a precooked packaged ham of topmost quality. These are not canned and will be found in the meat department. The price is high, but not as high as the boiled ham in the delicatessen section. It is as fat free as ham can ever be, so that your family can use smaller servings than usual. Buy it on sale, especially for company dinners, and you will be surprised how far ham you might have thought too expensive will stretch. A 5-pound one will serve ten people and they are almost laborless.

One of the great ways to save money is to do your meal planning around the meat sales. Over a few weeks, the meats on sale always vary; one week perhaps a leg of lamb will be on sale, next a rump roast, then a ham. The savings can run about 20 cents a pound. Over the long run, it would work out even cheaper than buying a side of beef—besides there's no leftover fat meat.

A general meat-cooking rule should be observed for all of you on this diet. All soups, stews, spaghetti sauces, and pot roasts should be cooked a day in advance. Chill overnight, and the next day you can remove all the free fat very easily. You simply cannot get the fat off when the liquid is hot no matter what trick you try to use. It will also taste better the next day. For some of you, another new trick will be marinating: letting your meat soak in seasoned liquid to flavor and tenderize it. If you have never done this, it will be a surprise to your newly developing taste buds. For you who have done this in the past, you will find that you really don't have to give it up. You who are used to cooking with wines will recognize the substitutes when you see them. Please do not change the recipe when, for instance, you see diet ginger ale and lemon. It takes both of them to do the job.

Almost all of the recipes in this chapter are unusual. That's why you bought the book, for flavor and excitement and gusto. If you feel tentative, start with the minted lamb loin, and then escalate.

MINTED LAMB LOIN ROAST

Lamb has been a gourmet delicacy for so long that even in the Old Testament it is mentioned for festivals—the meat of richness and love. Here are two recipes, both about the same but they are cooked a little differently. (Good-by, mint jelly.)

2 large cloves garlic
1 cup diet ginger ale
2 tablespoons lemon juice
½ cup fresh mint leaves, crushed
8-bone loin roast (loin chops not cut)

Slice the garlic clove into four little pieces. Take a sharp paring knife and insert it about 1 inch deep into the middle of each chop from the top. Move the knife sideways, and slip the garlic into the crevice. Mix the rest of the ingredients and marinate the lamb in the liquid 4 or 5 hours in the refrigerator. To keep costs down, always marinate in a pan that just fits your meat. For this a large dime store bread pan would do. Throw away the liquid.

Put your lamb on a roasting rack and insert a meat thermometer sideways—that is through the length and in the middle of the meat. Heat the oven to 325° F. and put in the lamb. Many people have a notion that lamb should be well done. You paid too much for this roast to lose half of it by overcooking. Cook it to the same temperature as medium beef (160° F.). If your husband is on the diet and is adamant about the well-doneness, do it the first time at about 175° F. and drop it about 5° every time you cook it. On the fourth try, just watch him enthuse by gobbling. Also, don't tell him of your successful put-over since when a wife wins one of these arguments she really loses. If you are on the diet, just give your husband the two end pieces.

One lamb chop equals 2 meat exchanges   146 calories
(Here is where I would ask my doctor about meat for milk substitutes, among others, most others.)

MINTED LEG OF LAMB

This recipe is almost like the recipe for Minted Lamb Loin Roast, and I included it for two reasons. One, legs are easier to find and cheaper than loins of lamb. Two, the instructions for barbecuing can be used for whole chickens, not marinated in mint of course, and other small roasts.

Double the recipe for the marinade for the loin. Insert the garlic. I'd double that, too, but that is up to you. To marinate this, use a deep pot, such as a large saucepan or pressure cooker. Just plunk the meat in, big side down, and marinate in the refrigerator for 8 hours. Don't worry about the shank, no one is going to eat it anyway.

For oven cooking, place the meat on a meat rack and follow directions for loin roast. It will of course, take longer.

The best way to roast meat is to barbecue it. It is the oldest way to cook, and preserves the succulence and flavor. Oven cooking is really roast baking. For this, and other roasts, you need a barbecue with a cover and a rotisserie. Build a good, large bed of coals; the fire should be at the rear. The meat should turn away from you, and the drip pan (use a throwaway) should be in front of the fire. This should take about 2 hours for a five pound leg. Use a metal thermometer (not a glass thermometer) if you have one, and insert it lengthwise into the heaviest portion of the meat. Do not let the thermometer touch bone or fat.

As this is a roast, just slice your allowable meat exchange.

ALL-AMERICAN POT ROAST

Here is a recipe for everyone, even the meat and apple pie and potato man (ordinarily not considered in this book) who likes his meat well done. It's on the approved beef list for heart patients and the leftovers are good for the do "without butter for lunch bunch" I described earlier.

5- to 6-pound boneless, tied, rump or top or
    bottom round of beef
1 tablespoon flour
Salt and pepper
1 cup Beef Bouillon (see Index)
¼ teaspoon garlic or onion powder or both
½ teaspoon crushed rosemary
1 teaspoon MSG

The roast should be unmarbled, that is, one expanse of shimmering red meat with at least ¼ inch of fat all around it and no threads of fat running through it. Pat the flour and salt and pepper on the outside. Don't worry about the flour, it's on the outside fat, which you are not going to eat anyway.

Preheat your oven to 500° F. If you are not sure that your

oven temperature control is correct, you can buy a little stand-up thermometer at the dime store. You need the temperature accuracy for the Astounding Standing Rib recipe even more. Put the roast in a shallow pan (a throw-away will do) and place in oven for 25 minutes.

In the meantime, mix the rest of the ingredients in a good heavy pot roast pan with a lid that *fits*. Move the meat into the pot roast pan, turn the oven down to 300° F., and cook covered for about 2½ hours. Check it now and then and don't cook it so much it falls apart.

The juice can be used for our Fat-Free Gravy (see Index). If you want to make the gravy immediately, remove the meat from the pan and set in warm oven. Strain the liquid and put it in the freezer; in about 15 minutes you should be able to get the fat off the top and proceed with the gravy.

Since this is a roast, just slice off your allowed meat exchange.

ASTOUNDING STANDING RIB ROAST

You are simply not going to believe this recipe, and your first reaction will be sheer fright at gambling with a standing rib roast like this. But your roast will be equivalent to that of the most elegant restaurant. The first time I saw it done was at the home of the friend who gave me this recipe. It was Christmas and the roast weighed 12 pounds. The oven door was glass and when it all started smoking at the end of the first half hour we were both in trauma, helped by her husband, who kept saying we were insane for attempting such a daring feat, especially at Christmas. Later, I tried it with a 5-pound roast, and friends have tried it, all with unbelievable success.

Any size standing rib roast, over 4 bones
Flour
Salt and pepper

Dredge the roast in the flour and seasonings. As we mentioned in the pot roast recipe, don't worry about the flour; it's on the outside, which you will not eat. Also, remember to buy a little dime store thermometer if you are not sure of your oven temperature.

Preheat the oven to exactly 500° F. Put the roast in a meat rack and roast it exactly 5 minutes to the pound for rare, and 5½ minutes to the pound for well done. Please do not let the smoke bother you. Of course, it will. Turn on your overhead fan and open a window. At the end of the 500° F. roasting period, turn the oven *off*. This is not a misprint. Do not, *do not* open the oven door now or for exactly 2 hours. The roast is now perfect. Remove to a warm platter.

If you want to make gravy, follow directions given for gravy in All-American Pot Roast (see Index). If you want to be a martyr, you can make Yorkshire pudding for the other people, and skip the gravy. You won't find the recipe in this book—for us, Yorkshire pudding is just a fond memory.

Eat your allowable meat exchange amount and don't eat the fat. Save the bones (see the chapter on bouillons).

ROASTING BEEF

There is an old public speaking axiom: "Tell them what you are going to tell them, then tell them, then tell them what you told them." So, here it is again. Please use low temperatures for roasting beef—300° to 325° F. The meat shrinks less, good for your budget; it is more tender and more moist, good for the eating. The approximate times are: rare, 18 to 20 minutes per pound; medium, 22 to 25 minutes per pound; and, well done, 30 to 35 minutes per pound.

And, after that, I really don't time meat that way. I only use those times for an approximation of how long before dinner to start the meat. *Please* use a meat thermometer. Insert it into the heaviest area of meat, in the center, and don't let the thermometer touch a bone. I've been using the same little dime store thermometer for 10 years, and it deserves a medal for all of the good meat it has helped to prepare.

Even ordinary rump roast can be oven roasted, but at an even lower oven temperature. Use the thermometer, set the oven at 275° F., and guess at about 45 minutes to the pound. Cook to medium beef on the thermometer. Slice thinly.

For meats that make good roasts consult How to Eat Meat chapter; no seasonings except salt (lots) and pepper are needed.

HASH

I thought hash was forever gone until I stumbled onto this method. Like Fat-Free Gravy, I'm really proud of it. It tastes better than pre-diet hash. Many of my non-diet friends are using this recipe just because it tastes better and is almost foolproof. Please do not omit the chilling—that is what makes the recipe work.

2 cups chopped leftover roast beef (I use the
    blender, low speed)
2 cups boiled diced potatoes
2 cups chopped onions
2 cups fairly strong Beef Stock (see Index)
Salt and pepper to taste

Mix all ingredients together; put in the baking dish you are going to cook it in. Pack down firmly with your hands and chill at least 4 hours. Preheat the oven to 350° F., and bake until hash is steaming hot all through and the top starts to brown, 45 minutes to 1 hour.

For one:

¼ of above	3 meat exchanges	219 calories
	1 bread exchange	68
	½ vegetable B exchange	18
		305

MEAT PIE

You should eat a vegetable A exchange with this. Biscuits have much more fat than other bread exchanges, so you should avoid a salad with an oil dressing on it. Try the Tomato, Cucumber, and Watercress Salad (see Index), as it will complement the Meat Pie. Have Fruit Salad for dessert (see Index).

½ cup chopped onion
1 cup sliced cooked carrots
1 cup cooked sliced mushrooms
1 cup cooked peas
2 cups diced leftover beef (not packed down)
Beef Bouillon (see Index) as needed
½ recipe biscuit mix (use 1 cup of biscuit
  mix rather than 2)

Use a deep 8-inch Pyrex baking dish. Toss all of the vegetables and meat together and add beef bouillon until it comes to the top of the mixture.

Roll the biscuit mix to fit the 8-inch dish. Put on the top of the mixture and bake in preheated oven at 425° F. until golden brown, about 20 to 25 minutes.

For one:

3 meat exchanges	219 calories
1 vegetable B exchange	36
2 bread exchanges	226
(includes 2 fat exchanges)	481

STEAK

I really didn't write this to give you a recipe for steak. You certainly know what kind of steak you like (within the limits at the front of the chapter) and whether you like it rare or what. I wrote it to tell you how to keep fat eating down and how to save some energy.

I had written a whole chapter on pots and pans and kitchens, but it was so boring I couldn't stand it myself, so I left it out.

Buy a little hibachi or barbecue for steak broiling over charcoal. You can't beat it for taste. Don't ever bother cleaning it. When the coals are getting hot, put the grill, cooking side down, over the fire. It might get a little crusty, but germ-free it is.

Buy an old-fashioned iron skillet. Put oil in it, heat it to smoking, cool it, and wipe it out with a paper towel. Repeat this about ten times—no one seems to know exactly. Do not now, or ever, wash it or cook liquids in it. It is only for fat-free browning. If it needs cleaning, use salt and rub like mad. (Get some male help.) You now have a "trained pan." You can fry steaks and other things without fat. For steak, just heat it up *very* hot, put salt on the bottom of the pan instead of salting the steak; throw on the steak and cook it fast, and as you like it. This works best with the thinner steaks as you can cook the steak so fast no juice will run out and wet the pan. (If it does, just start over with the oil and the heating.)

For thick steaks or for bad weather when you can't

use the hibachi (remember, you can put the hibachi in the fireplace) you are stuck with the stove broiler and the mess. Buy dime store cake racks for small meals and place over throwaway pans. The little racks will fit in your dishwasher, or will wash easily if you soak them in your dishwater. When they get too crusty, throw them out. Here is how to clean your oven:

1. Watch any TV commercial showing oven cleaners.
2. Wait for a cloudy day, turn off the kitchen lights, and don't wear your glasses.
3. Clean your oven just like the pretty lady on TV. Spray. Wipe. Rinse.
4. Don't look for little tiny spots. If you have a friend (?) who looks at your oven, replace her.

STUFFED FLANK STEAK

I have cooked this for years and years. The only change from the original is the reduction of fat in the dressing and the browning of the meat. I really cannot tell the difference.

1 onion, chopped
½ pound fresh mushrooms, cleaned and sliced
1 cup Beef Stock (see Index)
2 cups crumbled dried bread
½ teaspoon poultry seasoning
Salt and pepper
1½-pound flank steak
1 tablespoon safflower oil

Simmer the onion and the mushrooms in ½ cup of the beef stock until half cooked. Toss together with the bread and poultry seasoning and salt to taste. Let it sit about ½ hour and check for moisture. It should be moist, since there is no fat in the flank steak to moisten it. Add beef stock if necessary.

Spread the dressing over the flattened steak, leaving about ½ inch around the edges. Roll it up like a jelly roll, and fasten the edges with cocktail toothpicks; lace heavy thread through and around the toothpicks. You have to hold it together with your fingers and poke the dressing back in if it starts to come out.

Now, salt and pepper the meat and brown it in the oil in your Teflon pan at high heat. Use tongs, not forks, to turn it and brown it all around.

Put the other ½ cup of beef stock in a heavy pot roast pan: put in the meat, cover, and bake in the oven at 325° F. about 1½ hours.

For one:

3 meat exchanges	219 calories
fat—flank steak is so fat free you don't have to count the fat for browning	
1 bread exchange (½ cup dressing)	68 calories
Mushrooms—vegetable A	—
	287

A good night for a salad with French Dressing (see Index).

SWISS STEAK

I would double this and save some for lunch the next day. Start the day before if the meat is fatty.

1 pound round steak, 1 inch thick, cut in 4
    equal pieces
2 cups canned tomatoes and juice (read the
    label for sugar)
1 teaspoon onion powder
1 teaspoon seasoning salt
Salt and pepper
¼ teaspoon oregano

Pound the steak with a wooden mallet until you get tired or bored. Brown the steak in a Teflon skillet or a trained iron skillet, as I explained in the recipe for Steak, until it is brown.

Squish the tomatoes and juice through your fingers into a bowl and add the seasonings and oregano. Pour over the steak (change to another pan if you used the trained pan), cover and simmer about 2½ hours. Chill overnight and chip off the fat. Be careful of sticking as you reheat.

For one:
3 meat exchanges   219 calories
½ vegetable A exchange   —

BEEF STROGANOFF

This is one you have saved your fat for. I don't make Stroganoff as many people do. It's not beef stew in sour cream. Try my way. Use an Everyday Vegetable with this. A melon ball fruit dessert would be a perfect complement to this dinner even if it weren't on the diet.

½ pound fresh mushrooms
1 teaspoon paprika
1 teaspoon salt
Freshly ground pepper
½ cup grated onions
½ cup Tomato Sauce (see Index)
1 cup sour cream
1 pound top sirloin steak
Basic Plain Rice (see Index) or tiny egg noodles

Clean, stem, and slice the mushrooms. Put them in a saucepan, cover tightly, turn to simmer. There is enough liquid in the mushrooms that will come out as they start to cook. They will stew in their own juice. When just about done add the rest of the ingredients, except the steak and rice; keep hot but do not let it boil.

Cut the steak in ½-inch-wide strips across the grain. Heat your heavy trained iron skillet; salt the bottom. Get it very hot. Sear each piece of meat as rapidly as possible. Use long-handled tongs for turning—no fork stabbing, please. As soon as they are brown, but still rare inside, put them in the sauce for only about 3 minutes. Stir and serve *immediately* on the rice or noodles.

For one:

¼ of above	3 meat exchanges	219 calories
	2 fat exchanges	90
		309
	1 or 2 bread exchanges	68 or
		136

NEW ENGLAND BOILED DINNER

This is the easiest recipe in the book, all cooked in one pot. Use it for days when you need extra energy. Start the day before!

1 corned beef round (not brisket—too fatty)
4 large or 8 small carrots
2 turnips, cut in half
4 medium potatoes, peeled and cut in half
1 head cabbage, cut in quarters

Cover the meat with cold water in a large stew pot; bring to a boil and simmer about 4 hours until the meat is almost tender. I have found these rounds vary tremendously in cooking time. So if it takes an extra hour, it won't matter as you have started the cooking the day before. Chill overnight and chip off the fat.

Reheat and when boiling add the carrots, turnips, and potatoes. Cover and cook for 20 minutes. Lay the cabbage gently on top, and cook for 10 minutes. The cabbage should be a little crisp; most people overcook it. Serve with horseradish if you like.

For one:
Slice off your meat exchange
 3 meat exchanges   219 calories
 1 vegetable B exchange   36
 1 vegetable A exchange   —
 2 bread exchanges (potatoes) 136
            391

These potatoes cooked in the beef juice don't really need any butter, so here is a completely fat-free dinner. Whipped cream on strawberries?

BEEF, VEAL, OR CHICKEN GUMBO

1 pound of either beef, veal, or chicken breasts
4 cups canned tomatoes (read the label for sugar)
1 medium onion, chopped
½ teaspoon thyme
1 bay leaf
1 teaspoon salt
Pepper
1 10-ounce package frozen okra
Artificial sweetening (optional)
¼ cup minced fresh parsley
Cooked Basic Plain Rice (see Index)

Start the day before!
Cut the meat in cubes and brown them in your trained (see Steak) iron skillet. Put in a stew pot; add the tomatoes

(squish them through your fingers), the onion, thyme, bay leaf, and seasoning. Simmer until the meat is tender, about 2 hours for beef and about 1 hour for veal or chicken. Chill overnight and chip off the fat.

Reheat the meat to a simmer and stir often to keep from sticking. Add water if necessary. Add the okra and cook about 7 or 8 minutes. If you like, add a little artificial sweetener to taste. Add the parsley and serve with the rice. No fat, again.

For one:

¼ of above	3 meat exchanges	219 calories
	a little less than 2 vegetable A exchanges	—
	1 or 2 bread exchanges	68 or 136

MEAT LOAF

This is a 2-pound recipe, so there is some left for sandwiches.

¾ cup coarse bread crumbs (fresh bread)
⅔ cup tomato juice
2 pounds ground round (very lean)
½ cup chopped onions
1 teaspoon seasoning salt
1 teaspoon "Italian" seasoning salt
⅛ teaspoon garlic powder

Soak the bread crumbs in the tomato juice a few minutes, then mix all of the ingredients together with your hands. Shape into a cylinder 4 inches in diameter (so you can judge your meat exchange). Put into a baking dish and bake at 350° F. about 1 hour and 15 minutes. When you are ready to serve, mark the center with a knife. Then make another mark in the middle of each half and then another in each quarter. One of these slices (⅛) equals:

> For one:
> 3 meat exchanges   219 calories
> less than ⅓ bread exchange   22
> ———
> vegetable exchange—negligible 241

VEAL SCALLOPINI SAN FRANCISCO

This recipe title will probably ban the book in San Francisco, but when I lived there I used to eat in an Italian restaurant on Polk Street near Pacific. It was one of those long, tunnel-like restaurants with no decor, but the waiters wore tuxedos. I sat at the counter and watched the chef fix the most delicious scallopini I ever ate. This is an approximation of his genius, and if he understands the diabetic diet, I know he will forgive all.

1 pound veal top round steak, thinly cut (Do not use the thicker veal which has been put through one of those meat-murdering machines known as tenderizers.)
2 tablespoons safflower oil (use olive oil if you are allowed)
¼ cup diet ginger ale
¼ cup tomato juice
1 tablespoon lemon juice
1 large clove garlic, crushed
Salt and pepper
¼ teaspoon oregano
1 cup cleaned and sliced fresh mushrooms
1 cup raw baby peas
Spaghettini

Pound the veal with a flat mallet to get it even thinner. Get the oil very hot and brown the veal as fast as you can. Mix the liquids with the garlic, salt and pepper, and oregano and add to the veal. Bring down to a simmer. Add the mushrooms and peas and simmer 5 to 7 minutes. Serve immediately over spaghettini.

For one:

3 meat exchanges	219 calories
½ vegetable B exchange	18
¼ vegetable A exchange	—
1½ fat exchanges	68
	305
1 or 2 bread exchanges	68 or 136

AUTUMN VEAL CASSEROLE

This is a good family dinner. It is easy to make and if you have not been oversweetening your foods, the sweetness of the apples will be a delight to you. The dressing can also be used under a slice of center cut ham or in the little Cornish hens.

1 onion, chopped
¾ cup Chicken Stock (see Index)
2 Pippin apples, peeled and chopped
2 cups crumbled dried bread
1½ teaspoons poultry seasoning
Salt and pepper
4 veal chops at least ¾ inch thick

Simmer the onion in the chicken stock until about half cooked. Remove from the heat, add the apples, bread, and seasonings, and toss together. Let this sit a little while to see if it needs more liquid. Add a little more Chicken Stock if it seems dry.

Heat your trained iron skillet. (I rub both sides of the veal with fresh garlic.) Brown the veal quickly. Put the dressing on the bottom of a baking dish—it should be slightly moist. Place the chops over the dressing, and lay a piece of foil lightly over the top. Bake at 325° F. for about 45 minutes.

For one:

3 meat exchanges	219 calories
1 bread exchange (½ cup dressing)	68
½ fruit exchange	20
½ vegetable B exchange	18
	325

(no fat exchanges used)

VEAL RUMP ORLEANS

Ask your butcher to save you a veal rump. Veal seems, at the moment, to be "under the counter," and it's a perfect meat for us. Start the day before.

1 teaspoon salt
⅛ teaspoon each:
  cloves
  pepper
  allspice
  thyme
  sage
  garlic powder
1 4- to 5-pound veal rump
1 tablespoon olive oil (or other if you are not allowed olive oil)
2 cups Tomato Sauce (see Index)

Veal is so fat free it will not brown well without some help from oil. Mix all of the spices and rub them well into the roast. Heat the oil in a pot roast pan and brown the roast rapidly. Pour the tomato sauce over it and cook slowly on top of the stove, covered, about 2½ hours. Chill, chip off the fat, and reheat. The sauce is perfect over spaghetti. Use spaghettini.

For one:
3 slices, 4×2¼×⅛ each, equal
   3 meat exchanges   219 calories
SAUCE
   ½ vegetable A exchange   —
   1 or 2 bread exchanges   68 or
                           136

Look, no fat again. Real salad tonight.

BAKING OR ROASTING CHICKEN

People on diets, and people not on diets, complain that chicken is too dry. That may be true—any overcooked meat is too dry. The point of confusion seems to be whether it is "done" or not, and some folks confuse moisture with doneness. Chicken should be juicy, and the meat should be soft. If a chicken were undercooked, the rare meat would be tough. The answer, again, is slow baking, between 300° and 325° F.

Another thing is, you really don't have to use oil when you cook it slowly. Simply salt it, sprinkle on MSG and onion powder (or preferably, granulated onion), and bake it. Like turkey, it is done when it is brown and when you can squeeze the thigh to where you feel the bone. The easiest way to bake chicken is to use a chicken cut into quarters.

If you want to stuff the whole chicken, use a quarter of

the turkey dressing recipe in Holiday Turkey for Eight (see Index). Use the thermometer in the thigh, and bake at between 300° and 325° F. until the temperature is at the poultry mark on the thermometer, about 180° F.

I really feel stuffing a chicken is a waste of time, as you get so little stuffing (for the family, not you), and it is just as much work as stuffing a turkey.

ELEGANT CHICKEN AND ARTICHOKES

This is simple to make and impresses guests. It looks attractive on the plates and the flavors are delightful.

2 tablespoons safflower oil (use olive oil if you
   are allowed to)
4 halves of chicken breasts
Salt and pepper
2 cups drained canned whole new potatoes
1 cup drained pitted black olives
1 tablespoon lemon juice
¼ teaspoon marjoram
¾ cup diet ginger ale
2 packages frozen artichoke hearts, thawed

Use a large Teflon pan, preferably electric, with a good tight-fitting lid. Heat the oil and brown the chicken on both sides; salt and pepper as you brown. Remove chicken breasts from the pan and put them in the lid (so you won't lose any juice). Pat the potatoes dry and brown them in the remaining oil. Season with salt. Add the olives. Put the chicken over the potatoes and the olives, skin side up. Mix the lemon juice and marjoram with the ginger ale and pour over all. Cover and simmer on low heat for about 40 minutes. Take the cover off and add the artichoke hearts, turning each in the juice so that they will be well flavored. Cover and cook 10 more minutes. When you serve this, serve all of the olives to the guests, and your family. Don't waste your precious fat exchanges on olives.

For one:
¼ of recipe	3 meat exchanges	219 calories
	1½ fat exchanges	68
	1 bread exchange (potatoes)	68
	1 vegetable B exchange	36
		391

CHICKEN MARENGO

This is an adaptation from a classic gourmet recipe with the forbiddens left out or cut down. Challenge your friends to a blindfold test.

2½- to 3-pound chicken, cut up for frying
Salt and pepper
2 tablespoons safflower oil (unless olive oil is approved)
½ tablespoon arrowroot
½ cup cider
1 clove garlic, crushed
1 cup cut-up canned tomatoes
3 fresh tomatoes, peeled, seeded, and chopped
½ pound fresh mushrooms, cleaned and halved
Fresh parsley

Season the chicken with salt and pepper. Use your Teflon frying pan, add the oil, and heat until quite hot, 360 to 375° F. Fry the chicken until it is golden brown. Turn the heat to simmer, cover and cook about 30 minutes. Remove from the pan and put aside in the lid. Mix the arrowroot with the cider, dissolve, and pour into the chicken pan with the garlic. Simmer and stir until it thickens. Add the canned tomatoes. Bring to a boil and then add the fresh tomatoes and the mushrooms. Put the chicken back in the pan, re-cover, and simmer for 15 minutes. Garnish with fresh parsley.

For one:
2 legs or ½ breast. This is a small chicken.

3 meat exchanges	219 calories
1½ fat exchanges	68
¼ fruit exchange	10
vegetable A exchange (1 cup)	—
	297

CHICKEN WITH CURRIED PEACHES

Another no-fat main course with your rice covered with a yummy sauce. What a time for an avocado salad. One-fourth of an avocado equals 2 fat exchanges, and ½ fruit exchange. So if you have saved 2 more fat exchanges for the day, you can have ½ avocado. You could slice it alternately with tomato wedges, and sprinkle with lemon juice and celery salt.

Salt and pepper
4 halves chicken breast
1 tablespoon arrowroot
2 teaspoons curry powder
1 cup Chicken Bouillon (see Index)
2 tablespoons lemon juice
2 cups canned artificially sweetened drained sliced
　　peaches (save the juice)
Hot Basic Plain Rice (see Index)

Salt and pepper the chicken and broil slowly on the lowest part of your broiler.

In the meanwhile, dilute the arrowroot and the curry powder in some of the bouillon. Add this to the rest of the bouillon and stir over low heat until it thickens. Season to taste. When the chicken is done, remove from oven and add the lemon juice and peaches. Pour the sauce over the chicken, peaches, and rice and serve immediately.

> For one:
> 3 meat exchanges　219 calories
> 1 fruit exchange　　　40
> 　　　　　　　　　　　―――
> 　　　　　　　　　　　259

(Short yourself a couple of bites of rice for the arrowroot)

CHICKEN TERIYAKI I

Several recipes in this chapter include teriyaki. It flavors fatlessly, and adds just an edge of sweetness. I don't think you will get tired of it. Orientals have been eating it for centuries and they aren't tired of it. Also, teriyaki is "free" on your list.

1 cut-up frying chicken
½ cup Teriyaki Sauce (see Index)

Put the sauce in a flat throwaway pan. Add the chicken and marinate for 1 hour, turning with tongs about four or five times. Pour the excess in a cup and leave the meat in the pan. Put it in a 350° F. oven and turn it and baste it with the sauce about every 10 minutes. Bake about an hour.

By the way, chicken wings cooked this way, but quite crisp, make a marvelous, inexpensive finger food for parties.

For one:
BIG CHICKEN
    ½ breast equals 4 meat exchanges 292 calories
SMALL CHICKEN
    ¼ chicken or
    ½ breast equals 3 meat exchanges 219

CHICKEN TERIYAKI II

Salt
1 whole large fryer, not fat
½ onion, cut up
Celery leaves
½ cup Teriyaki Sauce (see Index)

Salt the inside of the fryer; put in the onion and the celery leaves. Just skewer the open end enough so that the vegetables will not fall out. Tie the legs and wings and mount it on your rotisserie. If you barbecue it, which is the best way, follow the directions for the fire and all in the Minted Leg of Lamb (see Index). If you don't have a rotisserie, use a roasting rack and place the chicken breast down. Set your oven at 325° F. and start brushing on the sauce right away. Baste with the sauce every 10 minutes. It will cook in about 1½ to 2 hours, and it should be brown. If you are not sure, take a paper towel in your fingers and gently squeeze the leg. If it is so soft that you could, but don't, squeeze to the bone, it is done.

Your food allowance is the same as for Chicken Teriyaki I.

STEWED CHICKEN—FARM STYLE

Here is just a good, old-fashioned, inexpensive dinner. Nothing needs to be measured, and it will remind you of those good old fattening food days. Cook the day before!

1 stewing hen, cut up (approximately 3½ pounds)
1 tablespoon salt
Pepper
1 carrot, cut up
Several celery tops
½ onion
2 bay leaves
2 cups sliced carrots
2 cups cooked noodles
2 cups cooked potatoes

Wash the chicken, put it in a stewing pot, and add water until it is about ½ inch above the top of the chicken. Add a tablespoon of salt, some pepper, the carrot, celery, onion, and bay leaves. Simmer partially covered about 3 hours, until tender. Chill overnight and remove the fat. Remove the chicken and strain the broth (no carrot that has cooked 3 hours is edible).

Bring the chicken and strained broth to a boil. Add the carrots, cook for 10 minutes, and add the noodles. Continue cooking until the noodles are tender. Prepare the mashed potatoes while these are cooking. Put the noodles over the potatoes with some broth. No butter, but not one more bread exchange!

For one:
½ chicken breast—this is a big chicken.

4 meat exchanges, either short it or get that milk substitute from your doctor.	292 calories
2 bread exchanges (½ cup noodles on the ½ cup potatoes)	136
1 vegetable B exchange (½ cup carrots)	36
	464

After that, a plain vegetable A, a plain fruit, and don't complain!

CHICKEN SHORTCAKE

This recipe is in here for that day when you can't stand doing without a food binge and yet want to stay within your diet limits. I wouldn't spend my exchanges this way. What I would do is give the biscuits to my family. I'd put my chicken on a piece of good toast, have a salad with dressing, and use the other bread exchange for Tapioca Pudding (see Index), with oodles of fruit over it. No matter which, serve the chicken with asparagus—they are perfect together.

½ biscuit mix recipe (8 biscuits)
2 cups diced cooked chicken (not packed down)
2 cups Chicken Fat-Free Gravy (see Index)

Prepare biscuits according to package directions. Mix the chicken with the gravy and heat. Pour over the split biscuits.

For one:
3 meat exchanges	219 calories
2 bread exchanges (biscuits include 2 fats)	226
	445

Also allow 8 calories for the arrowroot in the gravy. You can short yourself a bite of bread to make up the 8 calories.

HOLIDAY TURKEY FOR EIGHT

I don't know why I titled this as I did; turkey should be a staple food for dieters. It is tops on the accepted food list and when you need good meat for lunches there is certainly no leftover problem. The dressing is a company dressing, I guess that's why the title; it is also fat free and all of the goodies in it are on the list. Also, I'm going to tell some things about turkey that might make you like it even more than you have. Please always try to buy a fresh turkey.

DRESSING:

1 to 2 cups turkey stock made from giblets and
    neck, as you make Chicken Stock (see Index)
1 pound fresh mushrooms, cleaned and sliced
1 onion, chopped
4 cups crumbled dried bread
1½ teaspoons poultry seasoning
1 8-ounce can water chestnuts, drained and cut up
⅜ cup chopped pecans
1 teaspoon salt
1 12- to 14-pound fresh turkey

Heat 1 cup of the stock to a simmer in a large saucepan;
add the mushrooms and onions and simmer for 5 minutes.
Let it cool so you can handle it. Mix up all the other
dressing ingredients and add the liquid with the mushrooms and onions. Mix well with your hands; ten fingers
do a much better job than a couple of spoons. Add more
stock if necessary, taste for seasoning. Set aside for a while
to be sure it is not too dry. Add stock as necessary.

Pull the big fat pads out of the inside of the turkey's
pelvic opening, wash the inside and pat dry. Spoon in the
dressing. Sew the opening together with a large needle and
thread so the dressing does not fall into the juice while it
cooks. Don't use skewers. Put the extra dressing in the
large cavity between the neck skin and breast and sew it
also. Tie the legs together and tie down the wings.

Now comes the turkey lecture. I have heard many people, especially men, complain that turkey is too dry. It usually is, and simply because it is overcooked. It seems that

when a woman tests her turkey in the large part of the thigh (that's where we were taught to test, don't feel bad) and a little pink juice runs out, she reacts as if the juice were nuclear fallout. Even though the thermometer registers the correct 185° F. and she has exactly calculated the proper time, pop goes the turkey back into the oven. The big issue is to get that ½ inch of meat around the center of the thigh bone done, while 6 to 7 pounds of breast, two wings, and two legs turn into instant dried meat. For heaven's sake, forget it. Don't eat it. Use it later for soup stock. Do anything but sacrifice your turkey. Test in the breast; if pink juice runs out, then 20 more minutes should do it. If it is colorless that is fine, the breast *should* be juicy.

Probably this is one of the reasons people foil wrap turkey. It keeps the meat moist, which is all right if you want steamed turkey. It also throws off the temperature and confuses the browning. Of course, you don't have to baste, which is a bore, but you won't have to baste with this recipe either.

The second great delusion is cooking breast side up. Maybe that is so there won't be any rack marks on the breast, but we are in the eating business and not the catering business. If the turkey is roasted breast side down, as below, the back fat will baste the turkey for you.

Get out a flat roasting pan, the one that came with the stove, and a roasting rack. Rub the turkey with safflower oil, generously salt it, lightly pepper it, and sprinkle a tablespoon of MSG on it. Put the rack in the pan, the turkey breast down on the rack, and be *sure* the turkey is at room temperature. Heat the oven to 325° F., and roast 20 minutes to the pound. The turkey will be done and just for extras the oven will be so clean you can wipe it with a towelette.

Now take it out and as soon as you can handle it, put it on a platter. Turkey should sit ½ hour before carving to allow the juices to reabsorb into the meat. Put a little turkey stock in the roasting pan, put it in the freezer so you can chip off the fat. Measure your giblet liquid and the liquid in the pan. Make 3 or 4 cups of gravy according to the Fat-Free Gravy recipe (see Index).

The Holiday Pineapple Salad (see Index) goes beautifully with this dinner and has the advantage of being made in advance.

For one:

3 meat exchanges (slice according to list)	219 calories
½ fat exchange (nuts, you could leave them out)	23
1 bread exchange (½ cup dressing)	68
vegetable B exchange about	10
	320

FRUIT CURRY

This recipe is for six instead of four because the way the fruit works out, you would have an extra little fruit salad for two and that seems sort of silly. Anyway it's made to order for a company dinner for hot days as you don't need the oven on. All you need for the rest of the dinner are veal chops or chicken breasts broiled over a charcoal grill. Get thick veal chops, 4 ounces each raw (3 meat exchanges cooked). Don't forget to eat a group A vegetable that you prefer.

2 peaches, peeled and sliced
1 cup honeydew melon balls
1 cup cantaloupe balls
1 cup drained diced pineapple (artificially sweetened —save the juice)
2 bananas, sliced
2 cups diet ginger ale
1½ cups Chicken Bouillon (see Index)
3 tablespoons pistachio nuts
3 tablespoons seedless raisins (soak in warm water —pat dry)
1 tablespoon arrowroot
2 tablespoons curry powder (more or less, depends on desired strength)
Salt (optional)
Basic Plain Rice as needed (see Index)
½ cup fresh grated coconut

Mix the fruit and ginger ale and refrigerate for 2 hours.

Drain the liquid from the fruit, including the reserved pineapple juice, and add to the chicken bouillon. Simmer for 15 minutes and then add the nuts and raisins. Thicken with the arrowroot dissolved in a little cold water. Dilute the curry powder in some of the sauce, and add about half of it. Taste the sauce and keep adding curry until it tastes right to you. Add salt if needed.

Now this gets very pretty. Place a mound of beautiful white rice on a large heated platter. Put the fruit over and at the edges of the rice. Spoon half the curry sauce over the rice and the fruit and sprinkle the coconut over that. Put the rest of the sauce in a gravy boat. Serve the meat on the same platter, around the rice, and serve the vegetables in separate dishes.

For one (⅙)

CURRY SAUCE:

2+ fruit exchange	95 calories
1 fat exchange	45
	140

RICE

1 or 2 bread exchanges (If
you have two, eat the rice
for both—it's so good. Skip
one bite for the arrowroot—
5 or 6 calories)   68 calories for 1
                                                   136 calories for 2

Don't eat the raisins. Guests only.

GLAZED PORK CHOPS

This is reminiscent of those reddish-colored spareribs you get in Chinese restaurants. But those are appetizers and this is real food for dinner.

¼ cup Teriyaki Sauce (see Index)
2 teaspoons grated orange rind
¼ cup fresh orange juice
¼ teaspoon artificial sweetener
1 pound (4 chops) loin of pork (Buy only the
    kind of pork described in the front of this
    chapter or you will have to add a fat exchange.)
½ tablespoon arrowroot
4 drops red food coloring

Mix the first four sauce ingredients and put them in a flat pan. Marinate the pork chops about an hour, and pour the liquid back into a measuring cup. If it does not measure ¼ cup, add enough orange juice so that it does. Mix the arrowroot with the sauce and stir until dissolved. Add the red coloring. Turn your oven to broil and place the pork chops on a little flat rack on the pan you marinated them in. (I use dime store cake racks for broiling small amounts of meat; no big broiler washing.) Paint a good amount of the sauce on top of the chops and place as far from the broiler as possible. Paint on more sauce every few minutes and when brown on one side, turn over and repeat the painting operation. If they get brown before you think they are done, just turn off the broiler, turn the oven to 300° F., paint again, and finish cooking, about 40 minutes.

For one:
3 meat exchanges	219 calories
part of bread exchange	5[3]
part of fruit exchange	5[3]

229

MANDARIN PORK ROAST

This is beautiful to see when finished and makes a company dinner, easy to prepare, no problem for your diet, as you can just slice off your meat allowance, and envied by cooks who aren't on any diet. You can serve this with die-

---

[3] Short yourself a bite of bread and a bite of fruit to make up the calories.

tetic peach halves, filled with Catsup (see Index), with mustard mixed into the Catsup.

1 center cut loin of pork (remember your meat rules)
½ cup Teriyaki Sauce (see Index)
½ cup pineapple juice (artificially sweetened)
2 tablespoons grated orange rind
4 to 5 drops red food coloring
½ package unflavored gelatin

Trim the fat off of the roast down to ¼ inch. Mix the next four ingredients and put in a long shallow dish or pan that "fits" the meat, and marinate in the refrigerator several hours, turning frequently. Save the marinade. Put the roast on your rotisserie and cook at 325° F. at least 35 minutes to the pound. If you do not have a rotisserie, use a roasting rack, and cook fat side up.

An hour before it is finished, add the gelatin to the marinade and brush over the entire roast. Repeat this several times during the last cooking hour.

Eat your allowable portion:
1 fat-free chop equals 3 meat exchanges   219 calories

APPLE PORK CHOPS

I like to make this as the extra apple can be nibbled while cooking to make your food exchange come out evenly.

1 pound very lean pork chops, cut into 4 equal
chops
Salt and pepper
2 tart apples
Ginger

Cut as much fat from the pork chops as you can. Season
them with salt and pepper. Brown them in your Teflon skillet. While they are browning, peel and core the apples, and
cut four thick rings from each of the four halves. Rub a
little ginger on each side. Add a little water to the pork
chops, top each with an apple ring. Cover and cook over
low heat until tender, about 30 minutes. Eat the leftover
pieces of apple while you are cooking.

For one:

PORK CHOPS	3 meat exchanges	219 calories
APPLE	1 fruit exchange	40
	(including munching)	
		259

SWEET AND SOUR PORK

Don't let "Chinese" cooking and that long list of ingredients scare you. If you overcook this a little, it won't matter as it usually does with oriental foods. But it is sweet
and lovely. You can also make this with boned cut-up
chicken breasts if you want to save a little money.

2 tablespoons safflower oil

1 pound boneless, fat-trimmed, pork loin, cut in
¾-inch cubes

1 cup sliced onions (lengthwise, in crescents)

½ cup Chicken Stock (see Index)

¼ cup Teriyaki Sauce (see Index)

1 cup thinly sliced celery

1 cup seeded, cut-up bite-sized pieces green
pepper

¼ cup Catsup (see Index)

½ tablespoon artificial sweetener

2 tablespoons pineapple juice

2 tablespoons vinegar

¼ tablespoon arrowroot

1 8-ounce can artificially sweetened diet pineapple
chunks (save the juice)

1 small can water chestnuts (watch for sales)

Basic Plain rice

Put the oil in a Teflon frying pan, preferably electric, and brown the pork slowly at medium heat. Add the onions and stir until the onions have taken up the remaining oil. Add the chicken stock and the teriyaki, bring to a simmer. Add the celery and peppers and simmer about 6 or 7 minutes.

In the meantime, mix the catsup, sweetener, pineapple juice, vinegar, and arrowroot until the arrowroot dissolves.

Add the pineapple and water chestnuts to the mixture in the pan; when they are hot drain off the excess liquid and save it. Stir the mixture constantly, while pouring the arrowroot sauce over it. This will thicken: if it clings together it is too thick so add the leftover juice and/or pineapple juice just a little at a time until the mixture is smooth and there is a nice bunch of sauce left to pour over the rice.

For one:

3 meat exchanges	219 calories
1½ fat exchanges	68
1 vegetable B exchange	36
½ vegetable A exchange	—
½ fruit exchange	20
	343
Rice, eat both of your bread exchanges	136

STUFFED GREEN PEPPERS

2 large or 4 small green peppers
½ cup finely cut onion
½ cup Chicken Bouillon (see Index)
½ pound ground beef (fat free)
½ pound ground veal
Salt and pepper
Pinch nutmeg
1 egg, beaten
½ cup bread crumbs
Tomato Sauce (see Index)

Cut the peppers lengthwise and remove the seeds. Simmer the onion in the bouillon until tender. Add all of the rest to the bouillon and mix by hand. Fill each half of the peppers and put in a shallow baking dish. Pour about ¼ inch of water in the bottom of the baking dish. Bake at 300° F. for 1 hour. Serve with tomato sauce over them.

For one:

3 meat exchanges	219 calories
½ bread exchange	34
	253

1 vegetable B exchange equals ⅔ cup Tomato Sauce
Add calories as you use Tomato Sauce.
Be sure to add another vegetable!

MACARONI AND CHEESE

Everyone likes this and I have always made Macaroni
and Cheese this way, instead of using white sauce. There's
something gluey about a flour product cooked in another
flour product, school-cafeteria style. Serve with two vegetables and any fat-free salad.

2 cups uncooked macaroni (8-ounce package)
2 cups milk
Pinch salt (cheese is salty)
2 eggs
2 cups ⅜-inch cubes Cheddar cheese

Cook the macaroni per the instructions on the package.
While the macaroni is cooking, beat the milk, salt, and
eggs together in a deep Pyrex (or throwaway aluminum)
bowl. Drain the macaroni (don't rinse) and add it and
the cheese to the milk and egg mixture. (If you need more
milk, keep track of it so you will know how much milk
exchange you are getting. The milk should come just to the

top of the mixture.) Bake 30 to 40 minutes in a 350°F. oven.

For one:

3 meat exchanges (cheese and eggs)	219 calories
2 fat exchanges (comes in the cheese)	90
2 bread exchanges	136
½ milk exchange	85
	530

SPAGHETTI SAUCE

It's a good idea to double or even triple this recipe and use it for two or three meals. It's no more trouble to make three of it than one of it, and it will freeze well. This is made fat free, and what else would you eat with spaghetti but a salad with an oil and vinegar dressing?

1 pound ground beef
1 tablespoon salt
2 cans tomato sauce (sugarless) or 2 cups
   Tomato Sauce (see Index)
1 cup water
1 clove garlic, crushed
½ teaspoon oregano (that's a must)
1 teaspoon chopped parsley (not a must)
Mushrooms, if you wish

Start the day before!
Put the meat in a hot stew pot on medium high heat and cut and stir with the salt until the meat is nice and brown and crumbly. Add all of the rest of the ingredients,

lower heat to a simmer, and cook 3 hours. You may need to add water if too much evaporates. Refrigerate and chip off the fat before reheating to serve. Do not rewarm the sauce on high heat as it is inclined to stick.

For one:
¾ cup   3 meat exchanges   219 calories
1 vegetable B exchange   36
                              ———
                              255

Please use spaghettini for your 1
or 2 bread exchanges. The thin
spaghetti makes it all taste better.   68 or
                                      136

HOW TO EAT

Fish
ANOTHER FAT SAVER

I have a bias about fish that started during the depression. My father used to go fishing about three times a week. The Pacific shore was so full of fish then that he always brought back about one or two gunny sacks full, and most of it was mackerel. To make it worse, he built a smokehouse and we had an endless supply. As the only way my father would eat fish was fried—I don't care for fried fish and I hate mackerel.

Both of these problems worked out very well on the diet, especially when I got one of my look-it-up fits on fish and found some interesting facts. Many fish are so fat free that you can calculate your food exchanges and deduct fat exchanges to use elsewhere. I have noted this in each recipe. Mackerel turned out to be a very fatty fish, so you don't get a recipe for mackerel, and now I have a "real" reason instead of an old habit reason.

For fish that you just poach, bake, or broil with only lemon or other seasonings you may deduct 1 fat exchange for each meat exchange with clams, crab, lobster, salmon, shrimp, and swordfish. Bass, mackerel, oysters, sardines (canned in oil), all need fat exchanges added to them so it is better to avoid them. (This kind of list was not included in the meat chapter as all meats listed do not need fat exchanges added to them.)

Another interesting item I dug up is that fish are just not fried in gourmet circles. Sautéeing, poaching, baking, and broiling are "in." Frying is out. You are "in."

When you have found your best fish store buy what is fresh and has never been frozen. You might have to ask them which is fresh—they won't volunteer the information. But when you get your eye trained you will see the difference immediately. Try the Grilled Fish Steaks recipe with frozen and with fresh fish. It is really two kinds of food!

COURT BOUILLON

This is for poaching fish. It is right out of the gourmet's mouth, so to speak, and is the "in" liquid for the cooking of fish. This is much easier to make than the other bouillons and there is no point in making it up in advance. There is no fat in it; it is very cheap; and you can use the same pan to poach the fish in after you fish out the vegetables.

1 quart water
1 small onion
1 slice lemon
1 bay leaf
Celery leaves
1 sprig parsley
1½ teaspoons salt
½ teaspoon pepper

Combine all ingredients. Bring to a boil and simmer for 20 minutes. You can make the bouillon early in the day and reheat it or just go right ahead with the poaching if you make it at dinner time.

TROUT AMANDINE

This is a lovely way to cook trout, and also a good way to use the milk in your diet for gourmet cooking.

4 trout
1 tablespoon lemon juice
1 tablespoon onion juice
½ teaspoon salt
½ teaspoon MSG
¼ cup slivered almonds
½ cup heavy Chicken Stock (see Index)
½ cup milk

Rub the inside of each trout with lemon juice and onion juice. Sprinkle them with the salt and MSG, and then sprinkle the almonds inside the trout, equally divided among the four fish. Mix the chicken stock and milk together, heat to just below boiling. Place the trout in a lightly oiled baking dish, pour the milk and stock mixture over them, and bake for 20 minutes at 350° F.

For one:
3 meat exchanges (4 ounces raw. Half
   of 8-ounce trout is just right)   219 calories
1 fat exchange (almonds)   45
                                        ____
(⅛ milk exchange—shorten one of
   your milk exchanges by ⅛ th.)   264

If you have brook trout, you may deduct a fat exchange. If you have lake trout, you may not deduct.

CASSEROLE OF FILLETS

1 pound fish fillets[1]
4 teaspoons oil (whichever you are allowed)
1 tablespoon finely chopped onion
2 tablespoons lemon juice
¾ cup cider
Salt and pepper
½ tablespoon arrowroot
1 tablespoon minced chives

Arrange the fillets in a lightly oiled casserole. Brush the fillets with half of the oil. Mix the onion, lemon, and cider and pour over the fish. Salt and pepper them to your taste. Cover with the casserole lid and bake for 10 minutes at 350° F. Lift the lid and brush the tops with the rest of the oil. Re-cover and bake for 10 more minutes. Remove the fillets. Add some of the liquid from the casserole to the arrowroot, stir until smooth, and add this to the remaining liquid, stirring over medium heat until the sauce thickens. Add the chives and pour the sauce over the fish.

> For one:
> 3 meat exchanges   219 calories
> 1 fat exchange[1]
> ½ fruit exchange   20
> —
> 239

[1] See footnote on Enchanted Fish for fat exchanges.

ENCHANTED FISH

That means I'm enchanted, not the fish.

1 pound fish fillets[2]
Court Bouillon (see Index)
16 to 20 cooked asparagus spears (see Index)
2 cups Cream Sauce (see Index)

Go to your best fish store and pick out very thin, yet large in flat area, fillets. As these are very delicate you may have to cook them one at a time. Take your largest skillet and place the fillets in it so that each is separate, or use a smaller pan to cook them one at a time. Put enough court bouillon in the skillet to cover the fillets and simmer 5 to 10 minutes. The meat will turn from its own silvery translucence to white and when gently prodded with a fork it should flake. (This applies to all poaching.) Lift them gently out and place them on a slightly oiled baking pan. Put 4 or 5 asparagus stalks on each one, and pour ½ cup sour cream sauce over each. Place under a broiler until the sauce begins to bubble.

For one:
3 meat exchanges	219 calories
SAUCE:	
1½ fat exchanges	68
less than ⅓ bread exchange	20
	307
Asparagus, vegetable A exchange	—

[2] If you use halibut, you may deduct 1 fat exchange; for salmon, sole, or swordfish, you may deduct 2 fat exchanges.

GRILLED FISH STEAKS

4 fish steaks, 1 pound[3]
¼ cup French Dressing
4 tablespoons bread crumbs

Place the steaks closely together in any container that will allow you to use minimum amount of dressing. Pour the dressing over them and marinate for 30 minutes. Dredge the steaks in the crumbs. Bake on a broiling rack in a 400° F. for about 25 minutes. Baste with the remainder of the French dressing if they seem to be getting too dry.

For one:	
3 meat exchanges	219 calories
¼ bread exchange	17
	236

SPICY FRESH SALMON

1 cup water
½ cup white vinegar
3 to 4 drops artificial sweetener
1 tablespoon pickling spices (tied in gauze)
1 pound salmon fillets

Simmer all ingredients except for the salmon together for 10 minutes. Pour into a skillet and gently simmer the

[3] See footnote for Enchanted Fish for fat exchanges.

fillets for 10 to 15 minutes. Do not boil. Serve with Tartar Sauce (see Index) or Fish Cucumber Sauce (see Index).

For one:
3 meat exchanges   219 calories
1 fat exchange[4] Tartar Sauce

BROILED SHRIMP

Buy as many medium shrimp (remember that's large in the supermarket) as you are allowed or can afford. Clean, shell, and devein shrimp. Dip into Teriyaki Sauce (see Index) and put on a broiler pan. Broil until the meat turns pinkish white and starts to brown. Brush with teriyaki if shrimp start to dry during broiling.

Dip into Everywhere Sauce (see Index) when eating.

For one:
5 shrimp 1 meat exchange 73 calories
Add a free-fat exchange for every 5 shrimp.

FISH ORLEANS

1 whole 1¼-pound fish[5]
Lemon juice

[4] You have 2 fat exchanges for this amount of salmon. I counted 1 for the sauce, and you still have 1 to use elsewhere.

[5] If you use halibut, you may deduct 1 fat exchange; for salmon, sole, or swordfish you may deduct 2 fat exchanges.

DRESSING:

½ cup bread crumbs
¼ cup Chicken Bouillon (see Index)
1 teaspoon parsley
¼ teaspoon thyme
1 slice lemon, minced, including rind
3 tablespoons chopped cooked mushrooms

Salt and pepper
2 cups stewed tomatoes (break up with fingers)
1 teaspoon chopped onion
1 teaspoon salt
1 teaspoon minced fresh parsley
1 tablespoon arrowroot

Rub the inside of the fish with the lemon juice. Blend the dressing ingredients together and stuff the fish with them. Sew the edges of the fish together. Salt and pepper the fish.

Place the fish in a lightly oiled baking dish and mix the tomatoes, onion, salt, and parsley; pour over the fish. Cover and bake for 30 minutes at 350° F. Remove the fish to warm platter. Mix the arrowroot with a little of the juice in a cup and add that to the rest of the sauce from the baking dish, stirring over low heat until it thickens. Pour over the fish on the platter.

For one:
3 meat exchanges   219 calories
⅛ bread exchange (Short yourself
    elsewhere)   9
½ vegetable A exchange   —
                                                                  228

SCAMPI (SHRIMP)

20 large raw shrimp
4 teaspoons safflower oil (or olive if you are
    allowed)
2 tablespoons minced shallots or onion
½ cup Beef Stock (see Index)
1 tablespoon lemon juice
1 clove garlic, crushed
2 to 3 drops Tabasco sauce
½ teaspoon Worcestershire sauce
2 teaspoons A-1 Sauce

Peel the shrimp, devein, but leave on the tail. It looks
prettier that way and this dish can also be served as finger
food at parties. Put the oil in a Teflon pan and brown the
shrimp. Add the onions and sauté until they are trans-
parent. Add the rest of the ingredients, and cook 4 or 5
minutes. Put the shrimp on a hot platter and pour the sauce
over them.

For one:
1 meat exchange   73 calories
fat exchange (free)
fruit exchange (A-1 Sauce) (short
    your fruit exchange elsewhere)   8
                                         ——
                                         81

SUMMER SALMON

2 teaspoons unflavored gelatin
1 teaspoon dry mustard
½ cup water
1 teaspoon salt
1 egg
½ cup tomato juice
1 tablespoon butter
⅛ cup vinegar
1¼ pounds salmon steak
Court Bouillon (see Index)
1 or 2 cucumbers

Mix the gelatin, mustard, water and salt in the top of a double boiler. In a bowl, beat the egg and tomato juice. Add to the gelatin mixture in double boiler with the butter. Cook over boiling water, stirring, until the gelatin is dissolved. Take off the heat and slowly add the vinegar, still stirring. Chill until slightly thickened.

While the above is cooling, simmer the salmon in just enough court bouillon to cover, about 5 to 10 minutes. Cook until it flakes. Cool.

Peel and slice the cucumbers, and line the bottom of a pretty serving dish with them. Put the salmon over the cucumbers.

Take out the chilled gelatin mixture and beat with a rotary beater until smooth. Pour over the salmon and cucumbers. Chill well.

For one:
3 meat exchanges   219 calories
fat exchange (free)
fruit exchange (short yourself elsewhere)   5
                                                                        ———
                                                                        224

CLAMS AND EGGPLANT

Now, don't just go by this page. It is so different from
what you might think. And it has all kinds of advantages.
It is a fat saver; you get a lot of meat for 2 exchanges, in
fact, the most in this book. And you have a meat exchange left over for an eggy salad or dessert.

4 cups canned clams (save the juice)
2 cloves garlic
4 cups small chunks eggplant (see directions)
3 tablespoons minus 1 teaspoon butter
   (8 teaspoons)
2 tablespoons minced parsley
4 tablespoons minced green onions

Put the reserved clam juice in a large frying pan. Mash
the garlic and add. Cut up the eggplant, and drop it into
the clam juice as you cut it, as it discolors quickly. Add
the butter and cook for about 10 minutes, until eggplant is tender. Turn several times while cooking. Remove
the garlic and add the parsley and onions. Turn off the

heat, add the clams immediately, and mix well. Do not cook the clams, as they get tough.

For one:
vegetable A   — calories
vegetable B—negligible   —
2 meat exchanges   146
fat exchange (free)

                   146

HOW TO EAT

Potatoes, Rice, and Cousins

As I said, a baked potato used to be something you melt butter on, in order to hold up the sour cream. Almost all potato dishes that really taste good, from the ubiquitous French fry to the glories of gourmets, are all heavy fat users. Part of the sad story goes like this:

Baked or boiled, plain 1 small 1 bread exchange
(If you can eat this plain, I have only envy.)
Hashed brown ½ cup 2 bread and 2 fat exchanges!
(That is very poor—not really enough food to spend 2 breads and 2 fats each.)
French fries 6 (½×2 inches) 1 bread and 2 fat exchanges
(That's not enough to eat either.)

But there are many ways to avoid this problem. First, of course, use Fat-Free Gravy on mashed potatoes and life goes on just as before. Then, do not forget that in the Fat Food Exchange List 2 tablespoons of sour cream equal 1 fat exchange. This is sufficient for a small baked potato. Even better than that, several nationwide dairy companies make a sour half-and-half, which tastes just as good as sour cream. Three and one-half tablespoons equal 1 fat exchange.

Cook as many potatoes as you can in pot roast juice, stews, corned beef, so they get flavored as they are cooking.

Much easier than the fancier potato recipes are rice recipes. All you have to know is the Secret of the Orient, or how to cook it. After that, there are unlimited flavors that need no butter or any other oil. You can cook it in tomato juice, bouillons, onions and water, curry-flavored. . . . Potatoes just don't act this way—imagine potatoes cooked in tomato juice!

The secret is the pot. That's all. The pot must be thick, made from cast aluminum or iron, with a lid that is machined with a lip that matches the pot in order to obtain a steam seal. The size of the pot must be close to the amount of rice you are going to end up with. Rice expands four times while cooking, so if you start with 1 cup you get a quart. If you can't find the kind of pots described, try thrift shops. An old-time pressure cooker with a missing gauge is perfect for large amounts of rice.

Don't use instant rice. The labor is the same; measuring, cooking, and timing and the result is wet gluey rice that is twice as expensive. Plain rice is so obedient: merely use twice as much water as rice, cooked as below, and you always get flaky edible rice.

When you use spaghetti, use the thinnest you can buy. The taste, when whatever sauce goes on it, is entirely different. The thicker the spaghetti, the more canned it tastes.

With noodles, vary the thickness for the dish. Old-fashioned Stewed Chicken—Farm Style (see Index) just cries for thick noodles. Try the Fast Egg Dumplings (see Index) for this. They are halfway between a noodle and a dumpling, and make up in a twinkling, which is more than you can say for homemade egg noodles, if you have ever tried that. For dishes such as Beef Stroganoff, use either rice or noodles; the tiniest soup noodles are best. If you have good shopping facilities, try Chinese and Japanese noodles and Italian spinach noodles.

Just explore. Whether the noodles are farm style, Chinese, Italian, Japanese, big or small, you still get ½ cup for 1 bread exchange. Your explorations will solve the boredom of using that Food Exchange List as a cookbook.

BAKED POTATOES

For the best-tasting baked potatoes, please don't foil wrap your potatoes. They turn out partly steamed, flat-tasting, and they loose the texture that is unique to a baked potato. (If you want steamed potatoes, put a rack over water in a closed pot and steam them.) Scrub the potatoes with a brush, prick in two or three places with a fork, and bake at 400° F. for about 40 minutes. That is for the 2-inch potato on the list. Bigger ones take longer.

By the way, if you ever do have a potato explode in the oven, don't panic and do something like rushing the rest of the potatoes to a neighbor's oven. Turn the oven down to 350° F., wipe off the other potatoes, and finish cooking them. Test until they are done. Then, turn the oven to about 200° F., and cook the exploded potato until all moisture is gone. Cool the oven, and vacuum out the dry crumbs with the open hose end of your vacuum cleaner. No mess, no work.

NEW RED POTATOES

Please don't miss the short season that these elegant little potatoes are available. Clean them and boil them. Save some butter for these. Open them, butter them, add salt and a little paprika with some finely chopped parsley. When you buy these New Reds, be sure to keep them refrigerated as they will turn soft in only a couple of days.

POTATO CASSEROLE

4 potatoes, peeled and thinly sliced (2 full cups)
1 large onion, thinly sliced
Salt and pepper to taste
1 cup milk or more

Oil a deep casserole dish lightly. Alternate layers of potatoes, onion, and salt and pepper. Pour milk over all. If you need more milk, be sure to measure it. Divide the extra milk by 4; add this to your exchange. Bake in a moderate oven, 350° F., for about 40 minutes.

For one:
1 bread exchange   68 calories
¼ milk exchange   43
¼ vegetable B exchange   9
                          ———
                          120

BAKED HASHED BROWNS

This has half of the bread and fat exchanges of fried hashed browns. It is not a compromise, either; it is a truly old method of cooking potatoes, and it is a lot easier than hash browns that are fried.

4 potatoes, peeled and cut in ½-inch cubes
  (2 full cups)
1 large onion, coarsely chopped
Salt and pepper
1 teaspoon chopped fresh parsley
4 teaspoons soft butter (or margarine if butter
  is forbidden)
¾ cup boiling water

Mix the first four ingredients together. Put in a shallow baking dish about 1 inch deep. Spread the soft butter over the mixture. Pour ¾ cup boiling water over this. Bake in a hot oven, 425° F., for about 30 minutes or until the potatoes are cooked through and turned brown with a crust on top.

> For one:
> 1 bread exchange   68 calories
> 1 fat exchange   45
> ¼ vegetable B exchange   9
> ___
> 122

POTATOES AU GRATIN

2 cups finely diced peeled boiled potatoes
½ cup half-and-half cream
Salt
Pinch nutmeg
2 teaspoons butter
½ cup grated Cheddar cheese

Put the potatoes in a saucepan with the half-and-half, salt, nutmeg, and butter. Heat to a light boil and keep stirring until the potatoes resemble semi-mashed potatoes. Put them in a lightly ungreased baking dish, cover with the cheese, and bake at 500° F. until the cheese is melted. Keep a close watch at this high temperature.

For one:	
1 bread exchange	68 calories
1 fat exchange	45
½ meat exchange	37
	150

POT ROAST POTATOES[1]

Cook a pot roast, such as All-American Pot Roast (see Index), the day before you are going to use it and refrigerate it. Chip off the fat. Peel and cut 4 large potatoes into quarters and put them into the liquid. If necessary,

[1] You can do this with pot roast, stews, soups, bouillons, but never, never reheat an oven-cooked roast such as standing rib roast in this manner. It will ruin the meat. Use those meat leftovers for sandwiches or Hash (see Index).

add water to cover them. Put the roast on top of the potatoes and cook over medium heat, barely boiling, until the potatoes are done and the meat is reheated. Nothing needs to be added to the potatoes as they get lovely flavors from the juice.

> For one:
> 1 bread exchange   68 calories

POTATO BALLS

This is "rich," so eat these potatoes with one of the fish recipes where you get "free" fats. You still get more potatoes than if you fried them. I would reserve this for company, as you can start in advance, and it does have a bit of flair.

2 cups instant mashed potatoes (see directions)
1 egg
1 teaspoon celery or sesame seeds (try both ways)
Pinch nutmeg
Salt and pepper
¼ cup flour
1 egg yolk
Bread crumbs
2 tablespoons safflower oil

Make the potatoes out of an instant mix, using ¼ cup less liquid than called for so that the potatoes are much stiffer than usual. Cool until you can handle them. Beat the whole egg with the seeds, nutmeg, and a pinch of salt and pepper. Add the flour and mix until smooth. Add the potatoes and blend (use hands) until all is mixed well together.

Beat the egg yolk and put in a sauce dish. Make little potato balls with your hands. Roll the balls in the egg and then in the crumbs. Set aside for about 15 minutes. Put the oil in a flat baking pan and roll the balls in it until all are lightly covered with oil. Bake at 375° F. until they are golden brown.

For one:
Count how many balls you made. Divide by
4 and deduct 1.

1 bread exchange	68 calories
1½ fat exchanges	68
½ meat exchange	37
	173

MOCK POTATO SOUFFLE

I really tried to make a low calorie soufflé, you know, no cream, no thick white sauce; but I got very strange results. Potatoes have many characteristics; soft ones, crisp ones, wet, dry, grainy, and so this turned out not to be a soufflé at all; it's a custard. But I tried so hard, I was not going to give up the title. And I got a better potato recipe— and you couldn't be hungry after this—it is a real filler-upper.

16 ounces (1½ packages frozen) grated, not cubed, potatoes for hash browning
1½ cups warm milk, with
2 eggs, beaten into the milk, with
1 teaspoon salt, pepper, and good pinch nutmeg
½ cup grated onion

Let the potatoes thaw until they are at room temperature. Lightly grease a casserole, and put all of the ingredients into it. Stir very well. Bake at 350° F. for about 1½ hours.

For one:
⅝ milk exchange[2]	106 calories
½ meat exchange	37
1 bread exchange	68
¼ vegetable B exchange	9
	220

BASIC PLAIN RICE

Rice (and noodles, too) are so much more adaptable than potatoes that I think you will be very happy with all of the different juices and sauces you can pour over it. Pour Beef or Chicken Stock over it (see Index), use the sauces from meat recipes, such as Sweet and Sour Pork, Everywhere Sauce (see Index), and any juice you like. The simple fact is that rice can get wet and still be good, and potatoes can't.

2 cups water
1 cup rice
1 teaspoon salt

Boil the water, stir in the rice and salt. Turn the heat as low as possible and immediately put on the lid. Do *not* remove the lid while cooking. This should take 30

[2] I apologize about that funny-looking exchange, but that was what the recipe needed. All you really need to do is to throw 2 tablespoons of another milk exchange down the sink.

minutes. If the rice sticks to the pan, either the pan is too thin, or the lid does not fit well (see beginning of this Chapter) or the heat is too high. If it is the heat, use an asbestos pad on your burner.

RICE IN CHICKEN OR BEEF BOUILLON

Use either Chicken or Beef Bouillon (see Index). Use the same quantities of rice and liquid as for Basic Plain Rice. You can make any amount you want; always use twice as much liquid as rice, and after that anything goes. Add a little chopped onion, if you wish, and chopped mushrooms are excellent. A pinch of saffron is perfect with fish or chicken. Chopped fresh parsley is always good. You will need no butter on your rice.

ITALIAN BROWN RICE

2 cups tomato juice
Pinch oregano
½ green pepper, seeded and finely chopped
1 teaspoon salt
1 cup brown rice (not instant)

Boil the tomato juice, oregano, green pepper, and salt for a few minutes (in a thick pot). Add the rice and steam about 40 minutes. Besides your bread exchange, 1 or 2, short yourself a couple of spoonfuls of vegetable B exchange, for the tomato juice.

BROWN RICE PLUS

Try to find some short grain brown rice, if you liked the Italian Brown Rice. It's kind of earthy, and if you found plain brown rice earthy enough, just use it. This recipe uses fat, and is a nice show-off dish for company.

4 teaspoons oil (olive, if you are allowed)
1 cup brown rice
2 cups Beef Bouillon (see Index)
2 tablespoons chopped onion
1 teaspoon salt

Take the same old heavy pot, heat the oil over a fairly high heat. Add the rice and stir constantly until the rice starts to get more brown. Add the rest of the ingredients, and stand back when you add the liquid as it steams up quickly. Turn to low heat, cover, and steam 40 minutes. If you use short grain brown rice, it may take longer, but taking off the lid to check will not matter with this method.

½ cup   1 bread exchange   68
              ½ fat exchange   23
                                                   ——
vegetable B—negligible
                                                   91

RICE A LA INDIA

This recipe uses fat, and I would reserve it for company dinners. It is especially good with Mandarin Pork Roast (see Index).

2 tablespoons safflower oil
⅛ teaspoon artificial butter flavoring
½ teaspoon curry powder
2 cups cooked Basic Plain Rice (see Index)
¼ cup finely chopped fresh parsley

Warm the oil in your casserole dish. Add the butter flavoring and stir in. Add the curry powder and blend. Add the rice and the parsley and mix very well. Heat in moderate oven, 325° F., about 10 to 15 minutes.

One serving:
½ cup   1 bread exchange   68 calories
        1½ fat exchanges   68
                               ———
                               136

UNFRITTERED FRUIT FRITTERS

Breakfast, lunch, dinner? If you save fats, eat them for dinner. This is especially good with broiled chicken or either Chicken Teriyaki (see Index). The calorie price is high, but they are filling.

1 8-ounce can diet peaches, apricots, or pineapple (save the juice)
1 egg, beaten
¾ cup plus 1 tablespoon biscuit mix

Chop up the fruit as small as possible and mix with
the egg. Add the biscuit mix and stir well. Let it sit a
while to adjust for thickening. It should be like thick muffin
batter. Add juice from can if necessary. Use your Teflon
or heavy trained iron skillet at medium heat. Make any
size you like—smaller ones are easier to cook.

For one:
½ recipe 2 bread exchanges   136 calories
          1⅛ fat exchanges   51
          ½ meat exchange   37
          1 fruit exchange   40
                                ___
                                264

CORN FRITTERS

The calorie price is higher, so you get fewer.
Make exactly as fruit fritters, except use one 8-ounce
can of corn, drained, instead of the fruit.

For one:
⅓ recipe 2 bread exchanges   136 calories
          ¾ fat exchange   34
          ⅓ meat exchange   24
                                ___
                                193

I wouldn't bother with this unless on a very high calorie
diet.

FAST EGG DUMPLINGS

You can make them fast, cook them fast, and they are nice to eat, as they are so un-diet. Cook them in boiling soup, pot roast juice, or bouillon.

⅓ cup water
¾ cup flour
½ teaspoon salt
1 pinch nutmeg
1 egg, beaten

Add the water, flour, salt, and nutmeg to the beaten egg. Beat until smooth. Drop by teaspoons into boiling liquid, and cook uncovered for 10 minutes. Makes about 12.

For one:

3 dumplings	1¼ bread exchanges	85 calories
	¼ meat exchange	18
		103

PUFFY DUMPLINGS

This is higher in bread calories and lower in meat calories than egg dumplings. So choose where you want to be on your exchanges.

1 cup flour
2 teaspoons baking powder
¼ teaspoon salt
½ cup milk (try Chicken Stock, see Index, instead of milk, next time you make it)

Sift dry ingredients together. Add the milk, and stir until mixture is smooth. Drop by teaspoons into boiling liquid and boil for 5 minutes, *covered*. Count the dumplings and divide by four.

For one:
¼ recipe   1½ bread exchanges   102 calories
           ¼ milk exchange   43
                                   ———
                                   145

DIARY ENTRY 6

Vegetables and Mother

Things were improving every day. I was eating lunch as I explained before, and had already put together many of the meat recipes in this book—it wasn't a book then, the recipes were for me. But every night, I was forcing down the vegetables just like when I was eight or ten years old. Except then, I used to hide peas and things in my bedroom slippers.

As a graduate student in psychology I had enrolled in a class in Rorschach testing. We all had to take the famous ink blot test in front of the rest of the class, given by the professor, a gentleman of the old school. Mine went something like this:

ME: This blot is a frying pan.

PROF: Uhm.

ME: Here is a head waiter, with a tray.

PROF: Uhm.

ME: This blot is strawberries in whipped cream.

PROF: Show me the strawberries.

ME: They don't show.

PROF: Then how do you know they are strawberries?

ME: I know a strawberry in whipped cream when I see one.

Long Pause

ME: This blot is a baked potato and here is some hollandaise sauce.

PROF: Where is the sauce?

ME: Next to the two whole lobsters, where it belongs.

PROF: What color are the lobsters?

ME: Red.

PROF: They are gray on the card.

ME: They will be red when they're cooked.

CLASS: Snickering

PROF: Mrs. Meyer, you are a classified graduate student?

ME: Yes.

PROF: And not a comedienne? Yes?

ME: Oh, I didn't mean . . .

PROF: We will discuss your meanings in my office. Test discontinued.

In his office:

PROF: Mrs. Meyer, you seem to have some kind of problem.

ME: Oh no, I just think about food a lot.

PROF: And you don't regard that as a problem?

ME: No, you see, my mother—

PROF: Ah! Your mother!

(Mothers are the natural enemies of therapists.)

ME: —she always boiled all the vegetables.

PROF: Back to your comics! Mrs. Meyer, either you may discontinue my class or discontinue your insolence!

I just discontinued talking the rest of the semester. That "A" sure flew away quickly.

But I had insight! Those awful vegetables that my mother cooked were still in my subconscious. Dr. Freud would be so happy. Too bad I couldn't tell Professor X how successful his interview had been but I felt we had pushed the subject far enough.

I had but two alternatives. One: Psychotherapy, $40 an hour; Two: learn to cook vegetables, 29¢ a pound.

Maybe you have the same choice. First try my solution. It's cheaper. If you don't like my 29¢ choice, spend your $40 an hour after you have tried the vegetable methods and recipes.

Now that we've disposed of that problem, there are two other alternatives. There are two ways to cook vegetables. Elegant restaurants will invariably do one of two things. They'll serve vegetables with stark simplicity, scorning disguise or decoration. Or, they will go to the other extreme and have them practically unrecognizable under hollandaise or other embellishments. Here are the choices I have worked out for myself, starting with the basic everyday variety and working up to the more elaborate. There are two recipes for basic sauces (see Index). These can be added to almost any vegetable if you opt for camouflage.

HOW TO EAT

Vegetables

EVERYDAY VEGETABLES

Everyday vegetables means just that. Use this method for every day and use the special recipes for company or holidays. Use your energy on the meat course. As you will see, these vegetables need no butter for flavor.

Fresh Vegetables

Most of the non-leafy vegetables on the list are cooked the same way, but the labor is just the same as plain old boiling. The Chicken Bouillon (see Index) substitutes for the butter and the MSG brings out the individual flavor of the vegetables. As you know you are allowed 1 cup from the A list and ½ cup from the B list (in Appendix A) if your vegetables are cooked.

Amount	Time
1 head cauliflower, broken into flowerets	20 minutes
2 pounds summer squash (all kinds)	20
1½ pounds string beans	25
2 bunches carrots, sliced	20
20 Brussels sprouts	20
2 pounds (or more) tomatoes	10
2 pounds mushrooms	5

Artichokes (boil in water 45 minutes—there's no way out of it)

Basic Liquid

½ cup Chicken Bouillon (see Index)
1 teaspoon seasoned salt
1 teaspoon MSG
Pepper

A heavy saucepan with a tight-fitting lid is imperative, as the whole notion is to protest boiled vegetables. The lid is not to keep the steam out of the kitchen, but to cook the vegetables in as little liquid as possible. Add Basic Liquid to vegetables. Bring them to a boil, cover and simmer for the time given. Do not overcook—mushy vegetables have lost their soul.

Cooked leafy greens, spinach and others, do not need ½ cup liquid. Use 1 tablespoon of liquid and follow the method used for Sautéed Spinach (see Index). You can flavor these with lemon, vinegar, pickle juice, or Everywhere Sauce (see Index), all fat free.

Although I don't like canned vegetables—boiled, you know—I buy canned beets. What else can you do but boil them? Canned sauerkraut can be bought, too—what a waste of energy to make. Unless you can get really good tomatoes, buy them canned too, but read the label for sugar.

Frozen Vegetables

If you can't get fresh vegetables year round, frozen are the next best bet. Also on busy days, they save a lot of energy. But there is hope here, too. There's nothing really wrong with the vegetables, it's the directions on the package. If you follow those directions, guess what—boiled vegetables. Those directions are foolproof; you can't possibly burn them—render them unedible, yes, but burn them never!

Try this. Open the package at least an hour before dinner and thaw them. Then, change the basic liquid for cooking, and use that heavy saucepan and lid:

¼ cup Chicken Bouillon (see Index)
1 teaspoon seasoned salt
½ teaspoon MSG
Pepper

Cook the vegetables just about one-half of the time given on the package. I can't give you the exact time as freezing processes vary with different brands and that might change the cooking time. It's safe to do a little tasting here without deviating from your diet.

ORANGE HARVARD BEETS

½ teaspoon salt
1 tablespoon artificial sweetener
¼ cup vinegar
¼ cup beet juice
1 teaspoon freshly grated orange rind
½ tablespoon arrowroot
2 cups diced canned beets

Mix all of the ingredients except the beets in a saucepan. Bring to a boil slowly while stirring. Add the beets to the thickened sauce and heat slowly.

For one:

1 vegetable B exchange	36 calories
bread exchange (short a bite elsewhere)	8
	44

PICKLED BEETS

This can be a salad, or a vegetable, or a relish. That's a lot out of one easy little recipe.

2 cups drained julienne-cut canned beets
½ cup cider vinegar
1 tablespoon grated onion
1 clove garlic, mashed
Few drops artificial sweetener
1 tablespoon pickling spice (tied in gauze)

Mix, gently, all together. Let it sit in a covered container in the refrigerator for a few days. Remove garlic and spices before serving.

½ cup   1 vegetable B exchange   36 calories

OKRA AND TOMATOES

The okra both thickens and spices up the tomatoes without using up bread calories.

1 cup cut-up fresh or frozen okra
3 cups drained canned tomatoes (save the juice)
Salt and pepper

Cook the okra in the tomato juice with salt and pepper until almost done. Add the tomatoes and finish cooking the okra.

1 cup   1 vegetable A exchange   — calories

ESCALATED CANNED TOMATOES

For the winter solstice. Translation: the fresh vegetables are terrible.

2 cups canned tomatoes and juice
2 drops artificial butter flavoring
½ teaspoon artificial sweetener
1 cup *finely* chopped celery
2 tablespoons finely chopped parsley
Salt and pepper

Heat the tomatoes to a simmer. Add the rest of the ingredients and move gently about to mix flavorings. Cook only 5 minutes at a simmer so the celery is a bit crisp.

No calorie count
1 cup   1 vegetable A exchange   — calories

CABBAGE WITH APPLES

Fat free, good for home dinners, and overcooking won't hurt it.

1 medium head cabbage (red is prettier)
2 tart apples, peeled and cut small
1 onion, chopped
¼ cup Chicken Bouillon (see Index)
½ cup vinegar
1 tablespoon artificial sweetener
Salt and pepper
½ tablespoon pickling spice (tied in a square of gauze)

Shred the cabbage. Gently cook the apples and onion in the chicken bouillon for 5 minutes. Add the cabbage and other ingredients. Add water until the cabbage is covered. Stir again. Cover tightly and simmer 40 to 50 minutes. Drain excess liquid and remove pickling spice before serving.

For one:
1 cup vegetable A exchange   — calories
½ fruit exchange   20
¼ vegetable B exchange   9
                            ___
                             29

CABBAGE CASSEROLE

4 cups coarsely chopped cabbage
2 large onions, thinly sliced
Salt
Pepper
5 tablespoons flour
3 tablespoons minus 1 teaspoon butter (8 teaspoons)
   or margarine if butter is forbidden
2 cups milk

Boil the cabbage in salted water for 3 minutes. Put it in a big strainer and shake it until all water is drained. Lightly grease a casserole. Then alternate layers of cabbage, onions, seasonings, flour, and butter. Add the milk gently and bake at 350° F. for about an hour. If you need to add more milk, keep track of it. Serve this with ham.

For one:	
Vegetable A exchange	— calories
½ vegetable B exchange	18
½ bread exchange	34
2 fats	90
½ milk exchange	85
	227

SPINACH SOUR CREAM

Good to dress up frozen spinach and very easy. About the nutmeg: whole nutmegs are very cheap and they grate very quickly on your fine grater. Tastes entirely different from powdered nutmeg—use it in all recipes calling for nutmeg.

2 10-ounce packages chopped frozen spinach
½ cup sour cream
¼ teaspoon freshly grated nutmeg
Salt and pepper

Thaw the spinach and let the sour cream get to room temperature. Drain the excess liquid from the thawed spinach and put it in a saucepan with a well-fitting lid. Do not add water. After it starts to simmer, cook about 5 minutes. Strain out all of the water you can by mashing the spinach against the side of your strainer.

Mix the sour cream and nutmeg, salt and pepper, add to the spinach and slowly reheat while stirring. Do not let it boil. Serve immediately.

For one:
1 cup vegetable A exchange   — calories
1 fat exchange   45

ASPARAGUS

Asparagus and broccoli are probably the most mistreated vegetables served because no one pays any attention to the fact that it takes longer for the bottoms to cook than the tips. So if it is just all mixed up and cooked until the bottom is done, the tips are overcooked, and the tips are what you really bought them for in the first place.

(*For Four*)

2 pounds fresh asparagus
1 teaspoon MSG
2 or 3 drops artificial sweetener
1 teaspoon finely chopped green onions
½ cup Chicken Bouillon (see Index)
Salt and pepper

Soak the asparagus in cold water for ½ hour. Break up the asparagus with your fingers by snapping the stalks. As you get near the bottom, they won't break. Save these for soup and stuff—if they won't break, they won't chew. Use your large Teflon skillet, put in all of the above ingredients. Arrange the asparagus so that the bottoms are in the middle of the pan and the tips are all around the edges. If the asparagus is very small, don't break them up, but arrange them like wheel spokes in the pan, bottoms at the hub, tips pointing out. Bring to a quick boil, turn to simmer, and cook 10 minutes, then check. This can take up to 20 minutes depending on the size of the asparagus.

(*For Eight*)

4 pounds fresh asparagus
2 teaspoons MSG
1 teaspoon onion salt
1 cup Chicken Bouillon (see Index)
Salt and pepper

Soak as before but leave the stalks whole and just take off the tough end by snapping. Use a deep saucepan with a tight lid. (An old pressure cooker without the valve on is perfect.) Tie the asparagus together into a bunch with a string. Put the rest of the ingredients into the pan and stand the asparagus up in it. (If it tips over use crumpled foil around the edges.) Add water so that the liquid level is where the tip part starts. Spoon liquid over the tips. The tips are free of the liquid—they will steam done. Cover, bring to a boil, turn to simmer. Test in about 15 minutes. While the lid is off, spoon more liquid over the tips. Watch carefully if you need more cooking.

No calorie count for either asparagus recipe; vegetable A exchange only.

BROCCOLI

Broccoli is like asparagus in that the stems take longer to cook than the buds. But it is worse. You must peel the stems. My female friends who have observed this have either shouted with laughter or sneered at what they considered the finickiest eater of all time. But, to a girl, sometime or another later, they told me they, too, were peeling their broccoli. Peeling makes broccoli a delicacy, as the skins are both tough and bitter. Watch your children eat it once you have done this; at least that vegetable war will be over.

Cut off the stringy tough bottom with a knife, take a paring knife, and going toward the top just start to peel like an apple. It comes off just like a zipper—just a little pull and it will stop where the little branches start.

When you cook it, follow all of the instructions for Asparagus: for small amounts, stems in the middle of the skillet, and buds on the edges; for large amounts, standing up in the pot. The same amounts of seasonings and bouillon apply, except I put garlic in mine.

No calorie count for this; vegetable A exchange only.

BABY CARROTS FOR GROWNUPS

(*Actually the children will love them*)

When you can buy the smallest, freshest carrots on the market make this exquisite vegetable. It's a waste with big carrots. In "big carrot" season, it's time for soups and stews, as carrots are really two vegetables. The tinies are a gourmet's delight and the biggies add flavor to and take flavor from the longer-cooking dishes.

½ cup Everyday Vegetable Basic Liquid (see Index)
2 or 3 drops artificial sweetener
2 cups thinly sliced tiny carrots
2 tablespoons chopped fresh parsley (please don't use dried)
1 teaspoon chopped marjoram (¼ teaspoon if dried)
4 tablespoons heavy cream

Use a large, tightly lidded skillet and add the liquid and sweetener. Spread the carrots all over the pan. Bring to a boil, cover tightly, reduce the heat to a simmer, and test the carrots in 15 minutes. If they need more cooking, keep a close watch.

In the meantime, mix the last three lovely ingredients. When the carrots have just become tender, pour off any excess liquid, and add the herb and cream mixture. Mix them together tenderly—remember they're babies. Serve immediately.

For one:

1 vegetable B exchange	36 calories
1 fat exchange	45
	81

81 calories for this!

SAUTEED SPINACH

I don't know whether this is gourmet or peasant. Sometimes it's hard to tell the difference.

4 bunches fresh spinach
1 tablespoon safflower or olive oil (if allowed)[1]
1 clove garlic, mashed
1 teaspoon seasoned salt
1 teaspoon MSG
Pepper

Wash the spinach thoroughly in cold water, shake it out well, remove stems (very poor eating), and cut up the spinach into medium-size pieces about 2 to 3 inches square with a kitchen scissors. You can cut quite a few leaves at once and this goes very quickly. Put the rest of the ingredients in your large Teflon skillet, and turn

[1] If you are allowed meat fat, try making this with 1 tablespoon bacon fat, and omit the garlic. Calories are the same.

the heat to medium. Put in the spinach and keep tossing and turning with a wooden spoon. You should just about get the leaves covered with the oil when it starts to boil. Turn to simmer, cover immediately, and cook 5 minutes. Do not add water. Spinach is very wet, all by itself.

> For one:
> 1 cup vegetable A exchange   — calories
> ¾ fat exchange   33

BEAU TOMATOES

As I said, there are better places for butter than on bread, and this is one of them. These tomatoes are wonderful but do not waste one precious fat calorie on them unless you can buy the biggest, reddest, juiciest, top of the season tomatoes. If tomatoes such as these are not available, use the recipe for Escalated Canned Tomatoes (see Index) and save your fat calories for a good salad, or whatever fried memory you dream of.

4 tomatoes, as described
4 tablespoons butter (or margarine if butter is
    forbidden)
1 teaspoon MSG
½ teaspoon artificial sweetener
3 tablespoons minced chives or little green onions
2 tablespoons minced fresh parsley
½ teaspoon crushed oregano
Salt and pepper

Run very hot water over the tomatoes for a couple of minutes so that you can peel them easily. Core them with a sharp paring knife from the stem end. Put the butter, MSG, and sweetener in a pan and melt together. Roll the tomato tops through this and then place them core side down in the butter mixture; cover and simmer for 5 minutes. Turn the tomatoes over, and spoon the butter sauce over them. Mix the chives, parsley, and oregano and sprinkle them over the top. Cover and simmer another 5 minutes. Put tomatoes in a shallow serving dish, pour the rest of the sauce over them, and lightly salt and pepper.

For one:
1 vegetable A exchange   — calories
vegetable B exchange   4
onions negligible calories
3 fat exchanges   135
                          ————
                           139

Three fat exchanges seem kind of wicked, but if you live by the "How to Eat—Be Selfish" chapter, as I do, you have even more left.

MAGI ONIONS

For company dinner you can't do better than this. Few people will have ever had anything like it and it is a labor saver. You can prepare it hours before dinner and put it aside until 45 minutes before serving dinner. Cooks on top of the stove, too, so it saves oven space. Double it for guests.

20 small white boiling onions (raw, canned
    won't do it)

3 tablespoons safflower or olive oil (if allowed)
2 tablespoons vinegar
¾ cup diet sweetened plum, blackberry, or
 raspberry juice (yes, it used to be port)
⅓ cup raisins
Salt
Cayenne pepper to taste

Peel the onions; brown them gently in the oil (very slowly or else they will burn) until they are golden brown. Add all of the rest of the ingredients and cook at a simmer without a lid for 45 minutes. If you have no juice, and berries are in season, boil a cup of berries in a cup of water about an hour, strain them, mashing a bit, and sweeten with artificial sweetener to taste. You could also use unsweetened grape juice, which is always available.

For one:
½ cup 1 vegetable B exchange   36 calories
       2⅔ fat exchanges   105
       2 fruit exchanges (fruit
         juice and raisins[2]   80
                                    ———
                                     221

ITALIAN EGGPLANT

If you can't find mozzarella cheese, use California jack cheese. This recipe goes well with the Veal Scallopine San

---

[2] If you eat the raisins, you are being capricious. You and your guests aren't in the same ball game. Save the calories, the onions are good enough by themselves. Now, deduct 80 calories, only 156 calories now.

Francisco recipe (see Index), and as it has 1 meat exchange in it, you can cut down on that expensive veal needed for the scallopine.

4 very ripe large tomatoes, sliced
1 large eggplant, peeled and sliced
1 teaspoon salt
½ teaspoon pepper
½ teaspoon oregano
4 1-inch cubes mozzarella cheese
½ cup, or more, Beef Bouillon (see Index)

Use a large casserole. Put a layer of tomatoes on the bottom, cover with a layer of sliced eggplant. Mix seasonings and sprinkle one-fourth over the eggplant. Grate one of the cubes of cheese over the layer of vegetables. Do this three more times, ending with cheese. Pour the bouillon over until it is almost at the top. Bake 1 hour at 350° F.

For one:

	calories
1 vegetable A exchange	—
1 meat exchange	73
1 fat exchange (cheese)	45
	118

STUFFED ZUCCHINI

4 large zucchini
½ onion, chopped
2 tomatoes, seeded and chopped

1½ ounces grated Parmesan cheese (This does
   not need to be weighed. Commercial grated
   cheese comes in 3-ounce jars. Use half.)
½ cup bread crumbs
Salt and pepper
1 tablespoon chopped parsley
1 pinch oregano

Slice zucchini lengthwise and scoop out the seeds and
part of the pulp to make little boats. Discard what you
have removed. Mix the onion and tomatoes and simmer
them in their own juice until the onion starts to get tender.
Add the cheese, bread crumbs, seasoning, parsley and
oregano. Check the stuffing for moisture and add a little
water if it is too stiff, but don't make it runny or it will
fall off the zucchini. Put a little water at the bottom
of an open baking dish. Fill the eight boats with mixture,
and bake at 350° F. uncovered for about 20 minutes or
until tender.

For one:	
1 vegetable A exchange	— calories
¼ vegetable B exchange	9
½ bread exchange	34
½ meat exchange	37
	80

HOW TO EAT

Salads

Maybe you have a problem with your diet, especially if you are overweight, and when you have eaten what you are supposed to eat, you are still hungry. You know you should get a gold star for being a "good" patient, but gold stars aren't very filling.

The only way you can "overeat" on this diet is with raw vegetables, and that is one of the most important reasons that I have been constantly writing about saving fats. If you are one of those readers who just reads recipes and skips all the messages, go back right now and read the chapter entitled "How to Eat—Be Selfish," to understand fat exchange saving.

A *good* salad will fill your hunger needs, and a *good* salad needs dressing on it. If you were happy with a bunch of raw vegetables with no dressing, you wouldn't need this book at all. So, if you have saved those fats, you can still eat good dinners that are low in fat, and just go berserk with salads.

If you live in an area where fresh vegetables and lettuces are always available, the combinations of salad flavors are unlimited. Several kinds, iceberg, romaine, and butter lettuce, for instance, taste better than one kind of green.

You can use tomatoes one day (always take the seeds out as they dilute the dressing), onions another, thinly sliced cucumber, zucchini, or mushrooms, or little buds of raw cauliflower. You can change the recipe for French Dressing by changing the seasoning. The classic French dressing is made only with oil, vinegar, and salt and pepper, so you have no way to go but up.

How you prepare your greens is crucial. About an hour before dinner, wash the greens in cold water, shake the water off, and tear them up by hand. Chill them, and don't add the dressing until the last moment. Cold, crisp greens are as important as dressing. A little girl I know was taken to her first Chinese restaurant and refused the food, sobbing, "It's just hot salad."

There are recipes here for the winter months when fresh greens are hard to get. You can eat huge amounts of winter salads. Try the Sour Cream Salad Dressing (see Index), as you get more dressing per fat exchange. As you know, you may have 2 cups of cooked vegetable A, by omitting the vegetable B, and that's a lot of tummy filling.

And by the way, that old "gourmet" method of using an unfinished wooden bowl rubbed with garlic is *out*. The wooden bowl gets rancid, and also looks terrible after some use. At home use any big bowl and for guests buy a pretty glass salad bowl.

HERB AND GREENS SALAD

Practice with this to get the feel of a well-made green salad if you come from the old world of mayonnaise. Do not think I'm against mayonnaise; I love it, and if all of

the jars of mayonnaise I have eaten were laid end to end
. . . I really don't want to calculate it. It is too expensive
a fat exchange. One teaspoon of mayonnaise is simply
useless.

¼ cup French Dressing (see Index) (double
   if you have saved enough fat exchanges)
1 large clove garlic, crushed
1 tablespoon minced green onion
1 teaspoon fresh basil (¼ teaspoon dried)
1 tablespoon chopped fresh parsley
1 pinch powdered rosemary
¼ head iceberg lettuce
½ head romaine lettuce
Several sprigs watercress

Add all ingredients, except the greens, to the French
Dressing. Shake it well and let it stand a couple of hours.
Don't forget to remove the garlic.

Wash the greens, tear into salad-size bites (big), and
put into your salad bowl over several crumpled paper
towels. Cover with a dish towel and chill. Remove the
paper towels, toss dressing and greens together, and serve
at once.

For one:
1½ fat exchanges   68 calories

HIGH "C" SALAD

Don't be cowardly about trying raw spinach. Don't
tell and someone will say about halfway through his salad,
"Why, it's spinach!". The conversion is over.

1 pound spinach
1 large Bermuda onion
2 large or 4 small oranges
⅛ teaspoon artificial sweetener
¼ cup French Dressing (see Index) (double this
   if you have really saved fats)

Wash spinach several times with cold water to remove sand. Cut off the stems and throw away. Drain well. Tear the spinach into large bite-size pieces. Put a couple of paper towels in the bottom of your salad bowl. Put the spinach in the bowl and chill it well. Peel and slice the purple onion about ⅛ inch thick. Cut these in half to form separate little C's.

Have the oranges chilled. Peel them, separate them into segments, and pull off the membrane.

Add the extra sweetener to the French Dressing and shake it well.

Just before serving, remove the towels, add the dressing to the spinach, and toss lightly until the leaves are covered. Add the oranges and onions and toss about 30 seconds more.

For one:

1 fruit exchange	40 calories
½ vegetable B exchange	18
1½ fat exchanges	68
	126

COOKED VEGETABLE SALAD

In the summer, or in the winter, this is a nice way to eat vegetables, especially if you have trouble digesting large amounts of raw vegetables. Please read the section on cooking vegetables (see Index) and prepare them with Chicken Bouillon (see Index).

½ cup cubed carrots
1 cup ½-inch-length green beans
1 cup diced celery
1 cup cauliflower flowerets
½ cup ½-inch-length asparagus
¼ cup sour cream
¼ cup French Dressing (see Index)

You may cook the carrots, green beans, and celery together in salted water. Start with the carrots and add the beans in about 5 minutes, and the celery about 5 minutes later. Cook the cauliflower separately, or it will overcome all the rest with its own taste. Cook the stem ends of the asparagus for 10 minutes, then add the tip pieces and cook about 10 more minutes. Drain them all. Add the sour cream to the French Dressing and stir well. Toss the dressing with the vegetables while they are still hot. Be careful not to mash them. Chill.

For one:
1 vegetable A exchange   — calories
¼ vegetable B exchange   9
2 fat exchanges   90
                             ___
                              99

HOLIDAY PINEAPPLE SALAD

1 tablespoon unflavored gelatin
1 cup diet ginger ale
1 tablespoon lemon juice
½ cup pineapple juice
1 cup cottage cheese
1 cup well-drained crushed diet pineapple (save the juice)
1 cup chopped celery
40 almonds, slivered

Sprinkle the gelatin on the ginger ale and lemon juice; let dissolve and stir in. Heat the pineapple juice until boiling and add to the ginger ale mix. Stir well and chill until it starts to thicken. While this is chilling, put the cottage cheese through a coarse sieve. Mix all remaining ingredients and fold into gelatin mixture.

For one:
½ fruit exchange   20 calories
1 meat exchange   73
1 fat exchange (nuts)   45
                         ____
                          138

TOMATO, CUCUMBER, AND WATERCRESS SALAD

If you have no fat exchanges left for salad, this is a good combination, as the watercress is spicy and goes well with the tomato and cucumber. If you do have fat exchanges, don't forget to count them by the tablespoon, 1 or 1½ exchanges for the French Dressing (see Index), depending on how you made it.

Tomatoes
Cucumbers
Watercress
Lemon juice
Salt
Freshly ground pepper

Make as much or as little of this salad as you wish. Cut up tomatoes and seed them. Peel and slice the cucumbers. Tear up about the same amount of watercress as you use of cucumber. Sprinkle with lemon juice, season with salt and freshly ground pepper. Chill.

Vegetable A raw   unlimited

TOMATO DINNER SALAD

Easy and pretty. Here is a reminder on how to peel tomatoes. Actually I never bother. Turn on your hot water until it is as hot as you can get it. Run it over the tomatoes for about 2 minutes. (Don't believe instructions that give an exact time as each crop of tomatoes has its own personality.) Try to peel with a paring knife. If it doesn't peel, it isn't ready. Give it little dashes of water until it peels easily. Now:

1 cup julienne-cut cooked green beans[1] (see Index)
4 tablespoons French Dressing (see Index)
Peel and take out the seeds and sections of 4 excellent
   tomatoes

Toss the beans and dressing while the beans are still
hot. Chill, and stuff the tomatoes with the beans. Serve
on a bed of cold iceberg lettuce. You can garnish this
with slivered green peppers, sliced raw mushrooms, or very
thin radish slices.

> For one:
> vegetable A exchange   — calories
> 1½ fat exchanges   68

TOMATO AND COTTAGE CHEESE SALAD

(*For One*)

½ cup cottage cheese
1 tablespoon chopped dill pickles
1 teaspoon onion juice
Several drops artificial sweetener
1 tablespoon chopped watercress
1 cup quartered tomatoes OR
1 cup halved cherry tomatoes

Mix first five ingredients well and pour over tomatoes.

> 2 meat exchanges   146 calories
> 1 vegetable A raw   unlimited

[1] If you use frozen beans, you can purchase them cut in strips.

JAPANESE CUCUMBER SALAD

(*For One*)

Be sporting and try this. It's a grand fat-free way to eat cucumbers, and if you leave the fish out, there are no countable calories at all. But the fish really adds to it, so plan it when you are serving fish, and save 2 tablespoons for the next day.

¼ cup vinegar ⎫
Artificial sweetener ⎬ mixed to taste—sweet-sour
½ teaspoon MSG
1 tablespoon minced green onion
2 tablespoons shredded shrimp, crab, or salmon
¾ cup cut-up peeled, seeded cucumbers (quartered lengthwise and cut in ½-inch pieces)

Mix all ingredients except for the cucumber and chill for about an hour. When I make this for myself, I use raw salmon; it pickles in the vinegar. Try it. Add the cucumber and toss and serve.

½ meat exchange   37 calories

CHEF'S SALAD

This can be either for lunch or dinner, and is a good summer dinner. You have to do some fat saving in either case. The meats depend on your exchange for whatever meal you choose. "Julienne" means that you cut meats or vegetables in match-size (wooden matches, not paper) slices. As I said before, thin-sliced meats taste better, and "julienne" is such a beautiful word. Also, each salad is made in a separate bowl, so you can arrange your own salad for your diet, and make more for your voracious teen-agers or whatever. Of course, cutting julienne for teen-agers is absurd, so do it for guests or yourself.

Put as much chopped lettuce in the bottom of an individual salad bowl as you want.

For a 3 meat exchange salad cut

1 3×2×⅛-inch slice each chicken and ham and

1 3½×3×⅛-inch slice Swiss cheese into very thin julienne strips.

Arrange these around the top of the lettuce and put watercress in the middle. Place chilled asparagus tips around the edges, and pour French Dressing (see Index) over all. Assuming this is a dinner salad, this is:

$$
\begin{array}{ll}
3 \text{ meat exchanges} & 219 \text{ calories} \\
1\frac{1}{2} \text{ fat exchanges} & \underline{68} \\
& 287
\end{array}
$$

Or if you use 2 tablespoons of dressing, that is:

$$
\begin{array}{ll}
3 \text{ meat exchanges} & 219 \text{ calories} \\
3 \text{ fat exchanges} & \underline{135} \\
& 354
\end{array}
$$

CABBAGE SALAD

¾ cup Sour Cream Salad Dressing (see Index)
   altered as below
2 cups finely shredded cabbage

Follow the directions for Sour Cream Salad Dressing except use lemon juice instead of vinegar and omit the garlic powder.

Soak the cabbage in ice water, drain, and toss it around in a clean dish towel to remove the water. Mix with the dressing.

For one: 1 fat exchange   45 calories

IMPROVED CABBAGE SALAD

¾ cup Sour Cream Salad Dressing, as in Cabbage
   Salad (above)
1½ cups shredded cabbage
1 large apple, peeled and diced
1 banana, sliced

Follow the directions for Cabbage Salad, adding the fruit after the cabbage is prepared. Mix together and chill.

For one:
½ fruit exchange   20 calories
1 fat exchange   45
                     ———
                     65

VASTLY IMPROVED CABBAGE SALAD

¾ cup Sour Cream Salad Dressing, as in
   Cabbage Salad (above)
1 cup shredded cabbage
1 cup diced drained diet pineapple
1 banana, sliced
4 tablespoons raisins

> For one:
> 1 fruit exchange   40 calories
> 1 fat exchange   45
>   ──
>   85

This could continue to infinity. Any statistician will
tell you that if you took ten ingredients (add grapes,
celery, nuts, etc.) there are 3,628,800 ways of combining
them. You may finish the other 3,628,797 ways.

CARROT SALAD

This has got to be good for you. It's in every school
cafeteria in the United States. I still like it.

1½ cups grated carrots
4 tablespoons raisins
½ cup diced celery
1 banana, sliced
½ cup Salad Dressing for Greens (see Index)

Mix all and chill.

For one:
1 fruit exchange   40 calories
Salad dressing—omit ¼ of 1 whole
   milk exchange from this meal.

WINTER SALAD

1 cup drained canned pickled beets, chilled
1 Bermuda onion
1 cup drained canned pickled green beans, chilled
½ cup Salad Dressing (see Index)

Cut the beets in strips. Peel and slice the onion. Cut
each slice in half and separate the onion. Arrange four
equal parts of the vegetables on lettuce leaves (if any
are available) in patterns. Pour 2 tablespoons of dressing
over each salad.

For one:
½ vegetable B exchange   18 calories
Salad dressing—Omit ¼ of 1 whole
   milk exchange from this meal.

ASPARAGUS AND TOMATO SALAD

(*For One*)

There is something about grating an egg that moves it
from barnyard to gourmet. I don't know why. I would

eat this with hot sour dough rolls (unbuttered) for a fat-free lunch.

1 tomato, sliced
1 cup cooked asparagus tips (see Index)
Lemon juice
¼ cup cottage cheese
Seasoning salt
1 hard-cooked egg

Arrange the tomato slices on a plate with the asparagus around it. Sprinkle with lemon juice. Put the cottage cheese on the tomato, and sprinkle with seasoning salt. Grate the egg over the cottage cheese and serve.

2 meat exchanges   146 calories

ORIENTAL ADVENTURE SALAD

Go ahead and try it. If you can, get fresh bean sprouts; please use them, they are so easy to fix. Otherwise, drain and chill the canned ones.

3 cups bean sprouts
½ avocado, sliced as thinly as possible
½ cup cleaned, thinly sliced fresh raw mushrooms
4 tablespoons French Dressing (see Index—use
    the simple vinegar and oil dressing for this)

Pour boiling water over the fresh bean sprouts, drain, and then chill them well. Spread the bean sprouts on four salad plates, then arrange the avocado and mushrooms over that. Pour 1 tablespoon dressing over each salad.

For one:
vegetable A exchange   — calories
2½ fat exchanges   112

WALDORF SALAD

4 small or 2 large tart apples, peeled and chopped
1 cup chopped celery
2 cups drained diet pineapple chunks
4 tablespoons chopped walnuts
½ cup Salad Dressing for Greens (see Index)

Mix, chill, and serve.

For one:
1 fat exchange   45 calories
2 fruit exchanges   80
                     ——
                     125

Salad dressing—Short yourself ¼ cup whole milk from
this meal.

CELERY AND ARTICHOKES VICTOR

This is a fine salad for winter, or for company, as it is
made hours in advance.

1 medium-size bunch celery
Chicken Bouillon (see Index) as needed
1 package frozen artichokes, thawed
½ cup French Dressing (see Index)
8 strips pimiento

Trim the celery (about 4 stalks per salad, depending on the size of the celery stalks), string it with a vegetable peeler, and cut it up in lengths to fit a salad plate. Bring the bouillon to a boil; add the celery and artichokes. Cover and simmer about 10 to 15 minutes. Drain immediately and add the French Dressing while the vegetables are hot. Gently move the vegetables until they are coated with the dressing. Chill for 4 hours. Arrange the vegetables on the plate and decorate with the pimiento.

For one:
3 fat exchanges   135 calories
1 vegetable B exchange   36
                               ———
                               171

HOW TO EAT
Salad Dressings and Sauces

In a "gourmet" cookbook, sauces—all very rich—are usually the beginning of a recipe, and then another sauce goes over the top at the end of a recipe. Most of the recipes in this book make their own sauces as they are cooked, and in doing this, the "diet" as far as lack of flavor disappears and so do the rich sauces.

However, a few sauces are needed, and some are wanted, and some are new to you. Everywhere Sauce and Teriyaki Sauce are calorie free. Everywhere Sauce goes everywhere and Teriyaki is used in many fat-free recipes.

One of the most important reasons to save fat exchanges is for your salads to be salads, and the French Dressing recipe is for that, as is the Sour Cream Salad Dressing. There is also a recipe for fat-free Thousand Island Dressing.

If you can have enough fat exchanges to eat commerical mayonnaise, I don't think you are on this diet. But there is a Salad Dressing for Greens recipe, which is very low in calories, 122 calories for half a cup versus 890 calories for the same amount of mayonnaise.

Recipes for Tomato Sauce, Catsup, and Cocktail Sauce are here only because of sugar. For instance, commercial catsup is counted as 2½ tablespoons, equaling 1 fruit exchange. If you are allowed to eat the commercial ones, don't work.

Don't overlook the Fish Cucumber Sauce. It is really very nice on plain broiled or poached fish.

EVERYWHERE SAUCE—FAT FREE

I feel I have to convince you of how good this is because it isn't apparent from reading the recipe. It tastes different on different foods and is fast to make. Children love it, especially on those tiny egg noodles. It's good on rice and spaghetti. You can serve it in little sauce dishes and dip plain boiled shrimp or plain broiled fish. For parties, you can broil little meatballs in the oven, then keep warm in the sauce. You might try cooking string beans in it with mushrooms. You can try it on anything except, maybe, mashed potatoes—they get a bit soupy. But there is Fat-Free Gravy for potatoes.

1 cup strong Beef Stock (see Index)
2 tablespoons soy sauce
Few drops artificial sweetener (taste, do not get it sweet tasting)
½ teaspoon MSG
¼ cup grated turnip (if you don't have trunips, make the sauce anyway)
1 tablespoon finely chopped green onion or ½ teaspoon onion powder

Mix all, heat to a boil for a few minutes. Be sure to store any left in the refrigerator. It will spoil very rapidly but you can freeze it if you wish. This makes about 1¼ cups of sauce.

No calorie count

TERIYAKI SAUCE

Not only is this teriyaki sauce sugar free, and calorie free, but it tastes better and is cheaper than the ones you can buy. Make it in advance—I would double the recipe— and refrigerate it. It seems to last forever. It is used in many recipes in this book and you will find other ways to use it— marinate a steak, brush over barbecued hamburger. Try very hard to find fresh ginger; it too is cheap, is used in other recipes, will freeze in a little plastic bag, and tastes better by fourteen times.

1 cup soy sauce
½ tablespoon artificial sweetener
2 cloves garlic, crushed
1 teaspoon dry mustard
1 teaspoon MSG
2 teaspoons grated fresh ginger (1 teaspoon powdered)

Mix, shake, refrigerate. This makes a trifle over 1 cup of sauce.

No calories

FRENCH DRESSING

I've tried so hard and I just can't bring myself to do it. I can't make a good French Dressing that counts as 1 fat exchange for 1 tablespoon of Dressing, as your Food Exchange List says. Good French Dressing uses 3 parts oil to 1 vinegar or lemon. Prepared dressings aren't telling, I've read all the labels. So mine counts as 1½ fat exchanges, and is counted that way in all of the salad recipes. If you like a less oiled dressing, cut the oil down from 1½ cups to 1 cup, and you are exactly back to the food list.

In any case you should make your own salad dressing, so that you can eat your proper type of oil and control the sugar. This makes about 3 cups of dressing and takes about 5 minutes.

1½ cups light olive oil (if allowed) or safflower oil
¾ cup tomato juice
¾ cup tarragon vinegar
2 teaspoons onion powder
1½ teaspoons seasoning salt
1 teaspoon freshly ground pepper
¼ teaspoon dry mustard
1 clove garlic, mashed
¼ teaspoon artificial sweetener (more, if you
   like; taste after you shake)

Put all in a quart jar with a tight lid and shake. Refrigerate.

1 tablespoon	1½ fat exchanges	68 calories
2 tablespoons	3 fat exchanges	135
2⅔ tablespoons	4 fat exchanges	180

The simple way to make dressing, and the classic French way, is merely oil, vinegar, salt, and pepper.

1 cup oil
½ cup vinegar
Salt
Freshly ground pepper
The exchanges are the same.

SOUR CREAM SALAD DRESSING

This gives you more dressing with fewer fats. You can't improve on that idea.

1 cup sour cream
2 tablespoons vinegar
1½ teaspoons artificial sweetener
2 tablespoons onion juice
¼ teaspoon garlic powder
2 tablespoons finely chopped fresh parsley

Mix all of these together several hours before dinner and refrigerate so that the flavors merge. Don't make up too much of this at once, as it will not keep as long as French Dressing. This makes 1¼ cups of dressing.

3 tablespoons   1 fat exchange   45 calories

FAT-FREE THOUSAND ISLAND DRESSING

Personal choice is the issue on this dressing. You need to give up a meat exchange to eat it. But, for French Dressing you have to give up fat exchanges. Take your choice, or alternate, or toss a coin.

1 cup diced, peeled, and seeded tomatoes (if you
    can't get really good tomatoes, postpone this
    until you can)
1 large clove garlic
½ teaspoon salt
¼ teaspoon pepper
¼ teaspoon dry mustard
2 tablespoons lemon juice
4 or 5 sprigs parsley
1 cup cottage cheese
¼ cup dill pickle juice
2 tablespoons finely chopped dill pickles
1 egg, finely chopped

Put the first seven ingredients into your blender and blend until smooth. Pour into a container. Now, blend the cottage cheese and pickle juice until *very* smooth. Put all together, tomato mixture, cottage cheese mixture, pickles and chopped egg and mix together with a spoon. This makes about 2½ cups of dressing.

½ cup   1 meat exchange   73 calories
All other ingredients do not need to be counted.

SALAD DRESSING FOR GREENS

1¼ teaspoons unflavored gelatin
2 cups skim- or buttermilk
2 eggs, beaten
2 tablespoons vinegar plus 1 teaspoon artificial
     sweetener or 3 tablespoons vinegar[1]
¼ teaspoon pepper
¼ teaspoon salt
½ teaspoon dry mustard
1 teaspoon MSG
1 teaspoon celery salt

Soften the gelatin in a little milk. In one of your heavy pans, mix up the rest of the ingredients. Add the gelatin mixture and mix well with the rest. Stirring all of the time, bring it to a boil. Take it off the heat and beat well with a mixer or beater. Chill. This makes about 2 cups.

For one:
½ cup ½ milk exchange   85 calories
(you may add 1 fat for the day
without counting it)
½ meat exchange   37
                                                        ———
                                                        122

If you have saved fat exchanges, mix 1 tablespoon of mayonnaise to each half cup of dressing. You will have the closest dressing you can get that tastes like mayon-

[1] Vinegar alone makes a tart dressing. Vinegar and sweetening make a sweet-tart dressing. Do it to your taste.

naise yet have enough to make salads with. However, the total calories add up to 257.

SALAD DRESSING FOR MEATS AND SEAFOODS

Make Salad Dressing for Greens (see Index), leaving out the sweetener. For each ½ cup of dressing you wish, add:

¼ teaspoon salt
¼ teaspoon seasoning salt
1 teaspoon lemon juice
½ teaspoon cardamom (this is the most important ingredient)

Just mix the additional ingredients with the dressing. Make your meat salad in advance and chill with the dressing for several hours, for flavor exchange.

For one:
Same as Salad Dressing for Greens.

TOMATO, CATSUP, AND COCKTAIL SAUCES

If you can find any of the above already made, and purchasable almost anywhere *without* sugar, send me a wire, collect, and attain fame. Instead of that, I'll tell you about Italians.

Real tomato sauce, meaning Italian, does not contain sugar at all, and everyone makes his own. Canned tomato paste is about the only canned anything an Italian housewife would use. But we are not used to their kind of sauce

and are pretty used to that slightly sweet taste. So buy tomato paste, as it has no sugar (don't give up reading labels,
just in case). The Catsup, Tomato, and Cocktail Sauce recipes all have the same food exchange and calorie count—
but the seasonings vary. You can make two of these at once,
in different pans, and save time and energy. Be sure to
refrigerate them. If you want to use canned American sauce, you may use ½ cup of sauce, but it must be
counted as 1 fruit exchange, as it contains sugar. It is really
just what you want to do with your exchanges. I do it by
energy and not exchange preferences. If tired, I use
canned sauces, and skip fruits. But if I have time, I make
the sauces and enjoy my fruit exchanges elsewhere.

TOMATO SAUCE

6 tablespoons tomato paste (½ 6-ounce can—one
   reason to make two of these at once)
2¼ cups hot water
½ teaspoon onion powder
Pinch either marjoram, thyme, or basil
1 bay leaf (essential)
Salt and pepper
Artificial sweetener to taste (after cooking)

Put the tomato paste in a saucepan. After you measure
the water, swirl it around in the tomato paste can to get all
of that thick, thick paste out. Add all of the rest, stir well
and simmer without a lid for about ¾ hour, until you have
1½ cups left.

⅔ cup   1 vegetable B exchange   36 calories

CATSUP

This is also a fruit exchange saver. You may use 2½ tablespoons of this as a vegetable B exchange, rather than a fruit exchange, as purchased catsup must be counted. Two and one-half tablespoons of catsup on a hamburger sounds a little soggy to me, so if you use less, you have some leftover exchanges. Keep track of them, though.

6 tablespoons tomato paste (the other half of the can)
1½ cups hot water
3 tablespoons vinegar
½ teaspoon artificial sweetener
1 teaspoon salt
Pinch cayenne pepper
Pinch cinnamon

Put together as for Tomato Sauce. Simmer for 1 hour. This will be quite thick and will yield about ¾ cup.

2½ tablespoons   1 vegetable B exchange   36 calories

COCKTAIL SAUCE—ESPECIALLY FOR FISH

6 tablespoons tomato paste
1½ cups hot water
3 tablespoons vinegar
½ tablespoon artificial sweetener
½ teaspoon onion powder
1 tablespoon pickling spice (tied in gauze [imperative])

Make this exactly like the Catsup (remove spice after cooling).

2½ tablespoons   1 vegetable B exchange   36 calories

(Enough for a nice cold fish cocktail, or 5 lovely oysters.)

MARINARA SAUCE

This is more or less like the Italian sauces that are used more frequently than meat sauces. It can be used on spaghetti, rice, fish, poultry, and vegetables. It has few calories, and even though there is a bit of chopping, if you like it double the recipe. Please keep it refrigerated.

1 tablespoon safflower or light olive oil (if allowed)
½ cup finely chopped mushrooms
1 small green pepper seeded and finely chopped
1 onion, finely chopped
1 clove garlic, put through garlic press
1 cup Chicken or Beef Bouillon (see Index)
2 cups strained canned tomatoes and juice
Salt and pepper
Pinch thyme
1 bay leaf

Put the oil in a Teflon pan, and add the mushrooms, pepper, and onion. Cook over medium heat for 5 minutes, stirring with a wooden spoon. Add all of the rest and simmer about 1 hour, covered.

½ cup   ½ fat exchange   23 calories
The rest is vegetable A with a negligible amount of vegetable B.

CREAM SAUCE

This sauce is very light in calories compared to most cream sauces. It can be used where you would have used a white sauce for creamed vegetables.

2 tablespoons finely chopped onion
1 clove garlic, minced
4 teaspoons margarine
2 tablespoons arrowroot
2 cups Chicken Bouillon (see Index)
4 tablespoons sour cream
Salt

Sauté onion and garlic in the margarine for a few minutes. Stir in the arrowroot and blend. Slowly add the bouillon over low heat, stirring constantly, until it thickens. Take off heat and stir in the sour cream. Salt to taste. This makes 2¼ cups of sauce.

For one:
½ cup   1½ fat exchanges   67 calories
           less than ⅓ bread exchange   16
                                              ——
                                              83

PAPRIKA SAUCE

This is good on chicken and veal, and vegetables too. Make the Cream Sauce, but add 1 tablespoon of paprika to the arrowroot before you blend it in. Calorie and exchange counts are the same.

MUSTARD SAUCE (For Beef)

Make the Cream Sauce and add 2 teaspoons English mustard. You can use horseradish or other condiments as you like them. Calorie and exchange counts are the same.

CURRY SAUCE

Make the Cream Sauce and add enough curry powder to make it as you like it, but before you add the sour cream. Let it cook a few minutes, then finish as above.

WHITE SAUCE

If you prefer a more conventional white sauce made with milk, try this. The fat exchange is the same as the other cream sauces. The bread calories are very low, and it is a good milk user. You can make any other kind of sauce out of it by adding whatever seasoning you like, paprika, celery, but no lemon, of course, as the milk will curdle.

1 tablespoon butter
2 teaspoons arrowroot
1 cup milk
½ teaspoon MSG
½ teaspoon mild seasoning salt

Melt the butter and stir the arrowroot into it. Add a little milk, while stirring, until you get a smooth paste. Add the rest of the milk, gradually stirring until it just begins to boil. Add the seasonings. Makes 1 full cup.

½ cup	½ milk exchange	85 calories
	1½ fat exchanges	68
	bread exchange	10
		163

The calorie count is not as high as it looks as 85 calories include all or part of the milk you should drink anyway.

TARTAR SAUCE

This is much more fat free than a tartar sauce made with mayonnaise. Three tablespoons versus 1 teaspoon for 1 fat exchange!

½ cup Cream Sauce (see Index)
4 tablespoons sour cream
½ tablespoon pickle juice
½ tablespoon chopped capers
1 tablespoon chopped pickles (dill)
1 tablespoon minced onion

Mix and chill. This makes about ¾ cup of sauce.

3 tablespoons   1 fat exchange   45 calories

FISH CUCUMBER SAUCE

If you are short of time, try this quickie for a fish sauce.

½ cup sour cream
1 tablespoon lemon juice
½ teaspoon crushed dill
½ cup grated cucumber

Mix, chill, and let it sit and think. This makes about ¾ cup of sauce.

2½ tablespoons   1 fat exchange   45 calories

CRANBERRY RELISH

I've never seen a diet book that didn't have a cranberry recipe in it, so I'll conform. And, you need it for turkey, and . . . oh, let's be honest, I don't like cranberries.

1 cup cut-up, seeded, but unpeeled orange
1½ tablespoons artificial sweetener
2 cups raw cranberries

Use your blender. First, blend the orange until the big pieces are gone. Add sweetener. Then add the cranberries and blend until it looks like what you think relish should look like. This should make 2 cups of relish.

The whole recipe has 1 fruit exchange   40 calories
¼ cup   ⅛ fruit exchange   5 calories
                                          ——
                                          45

HOW TO EAT
Breakfast

I have tried very hard to find out what "the American" eats for breakfast. I polled my friends with these results:
> Soup, chili, aspirin and coffee, leftover chow mein, tomato sandwiches, coffee on the freeway, cold macaroni and cheese, doughnuts, wild rice.

None of this seemed to fit the list.

During a fit of insomnia I discovered an unrevealed sociological fact about breakfasts. The true breakfast habits are now an intense secret. While movies and books have exposed ALL, breakfasts are now secret—a new immorality. I know this because for 20 years I have worked in a "man's world" and in order to keep the fellows happy with a woman in their group, I feigned deafness so they could say what they wanted to. I have heard . . . well, they were probably lying anyway . . . but never a word about breakfast, sometimes dinner, but never breakfast. I know some of them must have eaten breakfast. How could they get so fat from only noon on?

Around my neighborhood the women don't eat breakfast either; they eat all morning. Betty goes to Alice's for coffee and doughnuts. Then, Betty and Alice go to Maureen's for coffee and coffee cake. Then Maureen has a snack with the milkman to keep current on Alice and Betty.

So who eats breakfasts as fictionalized in women's magazines. Several million diabetics. Everyone else is either lying or evading.

I'll just make my own categories as to breakfast-eater types. One, coffee and toast types, me, and, two, steak and eggs and potato types. For the first group, look at that breakfast! With just orange juice, milk, and 2 cups of coffee, you have almost a quart of things in the tummy and you haven't gotten to the meat and bread yet. For you type two's who are hard-working men there is no problem. Your doctor will give you a larger breakfast anyway, and you only have a problem with sugars. The recipe for Fruit Jam (see Index) will take care of part of that, and if you want to save fats for better dinners, there are recipes here so that you can do that.

For the rest of us, there is either too much to eat or not enough to eat. And either way, it's a bore. If you have been used to munching a lot of Danish, you think you are not getting enough to eat. The protein is important, so start with milk. Drink the whole glass of milk by itself. It *is* filling and has almost as many calories as an individual Danish. If you get tired of it, flavor it with artificial fruit flavors or brandy flavors.

For the coffee and toast crowd the best thing to do with the milk is to either make it part of the rest of your breakfast or talk to your doctor about a meat exchange for some of the milk.

To use the milk in the rest of the breakfast in the cold months, you can use it to make hot cereals. Use old-fashioned cereals, not "instants," and cook them according to the package directions; use either a double boiler or a controlled burner so that the milk will not boil. Experiment a few times until you get a consistency you like, and nothing needs to be added. Like cream, I mean.

In the summer, egg nogs and milk punches are good and can be made quickly. I have several recipes in this chapter and once you start making them you can make oodles of different flavors with real fruit.

If you get tired of this, try Egg Custard (see Index) for breakfast. You can make it the night before, so it's a morning time-saver. If your "sweet tooth" is really on, buy a diet pudding mix, again non-instant, that uses 2 cups of milk. Add 2 beaten eggs to it before you start cooking it, and when done, pour it into two bowls so you have two breakfasts. Count this as 1 bread, 1 meat, and 1 milk exchange. Pour Fruit Jam (see Index) over it and you have just eaten a 1500-calorie-per-day breakfast, and you have a fat exchange left over.

The 1 meat exchange (all breakfasts from 1700 calories per day down) is a problem. Bacon, of course, is a fat, and one piece of bacon is as silly as one peanut. Just forget it, and don't feel left out. People in the middle income group are only eating two slices of bacon a week each. Sausage is too fatty also, and you can only have one link, and that's as silly as one bacon.

If you can't have your milk exchange changed, the best meat exchange is the egg. Shakespeare must have had some kind of diet problem when he wrote "Thy head is as full of quarrels as an egg is full of meat." Just don't deep fry them in that good old hot pan of bacon grease. There are better ways to eat them, and there are a few recipes in this chapter. And a few ways to have a little meat, too, if you don't have leftover ham.

Also, use your fat-free griddle, either Teflon, or a trained pan, for pancakes. The recipe I have included uses very little fat, but you may use a mix if the box directions are "safe." "Safe" is low fat, both in them and how you cook them. In a packaged mix the recipe should call for 1 tablespoon of oil for about 10 to 12 pancakes. Just keep reading labels, you'll find one. One of these pancakes equals ⅔ bread exchange. Add ½ cup of Fruit Jam to the ones you make for yourself, and you have just made un-frittered fritters.

FRUIT JAM

A friend showed me this quickie recipe that turned out to be my breakthrough that made breakfast beautiful and saved that fat exchange for later. It can go on toast, French toast, pancakes, cereal, hot or cold. You can make it with apricots, peaches, pears, pineapple, all berries, such as blue, black, rasp, and straw. If you make it with apples, you get applesauce. It must be refrigerated. Don't double the recipe as it gets a little hard to handle with 4 cups of fruit.

2 cups any of above fruits
1 teaspoon lemon juice
½ envelope (½ tablespoon) unflavored gelatin
½ teaspoon artificial sweetener (or more if you want)

Cut up the fruit and put it in a covered pan over *low* heat. Do not add water. Check on it after 5 to 10 minutes, depending on the juiciness of the fruit. When the juice starts to come out, uncover the pan, turn heat to medium, and keep stirring until the fruit is about half cooked and a good amount of liquid has accumulated in the pan. Mix the lemon juice with some of the juice and dissolve the gelatin in it. Stir this into the fruit until all is mixed. Do not cook this until the fruit is mushy, as it tastes much better slightly underdone. Add the sweetener, stir, taste, and add more sweetener until it is to your liking. Refrigerate. Goodby, naked toast!

½ cup 1 fruit exchange   40 calories
(⅔ cup for blueberries)
(1 cup for other berries)

BANANA TOAST

This recipe and the next one are really meant for afternoon tea. So for afternoon tea, just have tea, and have good toasts for breakfast.

Toast both sides of a slice of bread. You can do this in either the toaster or the broiler; it's on for this anyway, and oven toast tastes different from toaster toast. Have ready sliced ½ small banana, and some cinnamon mixed with powdered artificial sweetener. Overlap the banana slices over the toast and sprinkle with the "sugar." Broil about 2 minutes or until the tops are browned a little. Serve hot.

1 bread exchange   68 calories
1 fruit exchange   40
                   ———
                   108

PINEAPPLE TOAST

Toast both sides of a piece of toast as you did for Banana Toast. Spread one side with 2 tablespoons *very well* drained diet crushed pineapple with a smidgen of grated lemon rind mixed in it. Sprinkle with the "sugar" mixture as in the Banana Toast recipe. Broil in the oven until the pineapple bubbles.

1 bread exchange   68 calories

Fruit—It is easier to short yourself 2 tablespoons of orange juice than figure the calories.

PINEAPPLE-HAM TOAST

I like to change the Pineapple Toast and add a meat exchange. Use the recipe for Pineapple Toast. After you toast the bread in the broiler on one side, put a slice of ham (1 meat exchange worth) on the untoasted side of the bread. Put this under the broiler for 1 minute, remove, add the pineapple mixture, and put it back under the broiler until it bubbles.

1 bread exchange   68 calories
1 meat exchange   73
                   ———
                   141

As in the Pineapple Toast recipe short yourself 2 tablespoons orange juice to avoid calorie calculations.

BROILED BREAKFAST BURGER

For beef lovers, here's a 1 meat exchange breakfast, juicy and good. Try it with sour dough or French bread or French rolls.

Toast one side of the bread in the broiler. Spread the untoasted side with 2 tablespoons (barely rounded) of very lean raw ground beef. It's easier to spread if the meat is at room temperature. Season with salt and pepper, and broil until the meat is a little brown and the juices are oozing. Serve hot!

1 bread exchange	68 calories
1 meat exchange	73
	141

THE PAN OF THE EGG

The point of all this is to save labor and also end up with eggs that taste like eggs.

Get a little cast iron, or a little copper-bottomed pan. The side of the pan should not have a corner with the bottom—it should be rounded, like a C. Oil it well, heat to medium hot, cool. Remove oil with a paper towel. Rub with salt if there are any brown grease spots. Repeat this process several times.

Keep this little pan for eggs only. Never, never cook liquid in it, never wash it, and never use it over medium heat. Use salt to clean it.

All you will need for scrambled eggs or open-faced eggs (formerly known as fried eggs) is 1 drop of oil on the end of your finger; rub it around, heat to medium; the egg will come out as you like it, leaving a clean pan. For open-faced eggs, cover while cooking.

PLAIN ONE-EGG OMELET

Please learn to cook your egg this way, rather than scrambled, because you get more egg, no matter what the laws of matter say.

Beat the egg lightly with a fork with salt and 2 teaspoons of milk (out of your allowance). Use the pan described above or a Teflon pan. Use medium heat only, and be sure the pan is heated before you pour in the egg. Pour in the egg and let egg settle a bit. When you see it start to firm up around the edges, tilt the pan while lifting the edge of the egg with a fork, and let uncooked part fill the space where you have lifted. Lift the other side and do the same thing. Repeat this until there is no runny egg left. Turn the whole omelet over with a spatula for about half a minute. Fold in half and serve. Now, you can see why you should train a pan, as your Teflon pan will get fork scratches on it.

1 meat exchange   73 calories

JELLY OMELET

Prepare the egg as in Plain One-Egg Omelet, and in the fold, put a couple tablespoons of Fruit Jam (see Index). Deduct 2 tablespoons of fruit from your orange juice.

CODDLED EGGS

I didn't used to eat coddled eggs, but when they cover the unbuttered toast, they take on allure.

Bring water to a boil in a saucepan. Lower the egg or eggs into the water with a tablespoon. Immediately cover the pan and remove from the heat. It takes 4 to 6 minutes for soft-coddled eggs.

1 meat exchange   73 calories

POACHED EGGS

Take a little skillet (not your trained pan) or a dime store poacher, and put enough water in to cover the egg. The yolk should be under the water. Add a pinch of salt. Bring the water to a boil, then reduce to a simmer. Break the egg into a saucer, and slide the egg into the water. Cover the pan and cook 3 to 5 minutes. Lift out with a slotted spoon or spatula, so the eggs can drain. Serve on toast or one-half of a warm English muffin. Season to taste.

1 meat exchange   73 calories
1 bread exchange   68
                    ———
                    141

POACHED EGGS IN MILK

Follow the recipe for Poached Eggs except use milk. Measure your milk exchange and pour out the amount you need to cook the eggs. Bring to a simmer, do not boil the milk. Put the poached egg on the toast and pour the milk over it all.

                1 meat exchange   73 calories
                1 bread exchange   68
                                     ‾‾‾
                                     141

DIRTY EGGS

On one of my wilder days I tried this experiment and now I eat it all the time. You will understand the title when you see it cooked. It's unphotographable. Don't serve it to anyone without warning them. Try it yourself first as the flavor is unbelievable.

1 tablespoon Beef Stock (see Index)
1 egg, beaten

Put the stock in a little skillet (not your trained pan) and on medium heat, bring it to a boil. Stir in the egg, and keep stirring until it firms up.

                1 meat exchange   73 calories

PUEBLO OMELET

I didn't have enough nerve to call it "Denver." This recipe is for people who have 2 meat exchanges for breakfast, and it is also a good lunch dish.

2 tablespoons Beef Stock (see Index)
1 tablespoon minced onion
1 leftover meat exchange (ham is best), minced
½ cup chopped boiled potato
Salt and pepper
1 egg, beaten

Put the stock in a small Teflon skillet and bring it to a simmer. Add the onion, and cook about 5 minutes. Add the minced meat and the potato and stir gently until they are quite hot. Taste for seasoning—the stock is already salty. Pour the egg over and keep turning gently until the eggs firm. Serve immediately.

2 meat exchanges	146 calories
1 bread exchange	68
	214

B vegetable—negligible

EGGS ARNOLD

Before your diet, you could have Eggs Benedict. Leaving out the hollandaise sauce is traitorous to a classic recipe, hence "Eggs Arnold."

Chop up a few fresh mushrooms and cook them in 2 tablespoons of Beef Bouillon (see Index). Poach a medium egg (see Poached Eggs). While poaching, take a slice of ham from one of the packaged super-thin sandwich hams. (They come in 3-ounce packages and one slice is less than ⅓ meat exchange.) Put the ham on one half of an English muffin, and place under a medium broiler (lower the oven rack if your oven is electric) until the ham and the muffin are hot. Put the egg on the ham on the muffin, and pour the mushrooms over the top.

1 meat exchange (ham and egg)	73 calories
1 bread exchange	68
	141
Mushrooms	—

SUNDAY EGGS

Every one in the family will love these eggs. The two-egg people can have two—I'm giving the recipe for one, as that is how you will fix them, no matter how many you do. Medium eggs are called for as they are a little less than 1 meat exchange and the cheese makes up for the rest. It is *not* a fat-free breakfast.

1 tablespoon heavy cream
1 medium egg
Salt
2 teaspoons grated Parmesan cheese

Use a Teflon muffin pan. Put the cream in each pan you want an egg for, break the egg into the cream and sprinkle the salt, then the cheese on top. Bake in a 350° F. oven for about 10 minutes.

1 meat exchange	73 calories
1 fat exchange	45
	118

Add a hot roll, a glass of orange juice, your milk, and there is a 1500-calorie-column breakfast, right off the list.

BASIC EGG NOG

With a blender, these whip up in a couple of minutes. Add any kind of artificial flavoring, brandy, strawberry—there's a myriad of them. If you use cocoa (unsweetened), you must add 30 bread exchange calories for each table-spoon.

1 egg
¾ cup milk plus 3 tablespoons fat-free dry milk
¼ teaspoon artificial sweetener
Pinch salt
3 drops vanilla
Pinch nutmeg

Put it all but the dry milk in the blender and blend 1 minute at high speed. Add the dry milk and blend 2 more minutes.

1 meat exchange	73 calories
1 milk exchange	170
	243

If you eat one of the solid fruit exchanges and a hot roll, you have a fat exchange saving and a breakfast from the 1500-calorie-a-day list.

FRUIT EGG NOG

Follow the above recipe, and omit the artificial sweetener. Add ½ cup of Fruit Jam (see Index) to the first blending. Add 1 hot roll for the 1500-calorie-a-day breakfast. Easy, isn't it?

BANANA EGG NOG

If you make this, you can add your other ½ cup of milk to ¾ cup of your favorite dry cereal, and you are still on the 1500 list.

½ cup milk
1 egg
½ banana
Several drops lemon juice

Blend for 5 minutes.

BUTTERMILK PANCAKES

Either use a trained pan or a Teflon griddle for these so you do not need to add fat.

1 egg, beaten
1¼ cups buttermilk
2 tablespoons oil (your proper type)
1¼ cups sifted flour
½ teaspoon baking soda
½ teaspoon salt
1 teaspoon baking powder

Mix first three ingredients. Sift together the next four ingredients. Put all together and beat with a rotary beater until smooth. (You can do all of this the night before by leaving out the baking powder and adding it in the morning. Refrigerate, and be sure to beat the baking powder in well.) Make 3-inch pancakes for yourself, and whatever size you wish for the rest of the family.

2 3-inch pancakes   1 bread exchange   68 calories

HOW TO EAT
Lunch

The easiest way to handle lunch on this diet is just not to make a big issue of it, especially if you want to save fat exchanges. I took another survey—this one at home. The lunch chapter of a famous cookbook yielded the following:

Of the 43 recipes in the lunch chapter
26 are completely out, and not even adaptable
 9 are fine
 8 are already in this book, one place or another.

Almost all of them are just *too* much work. Housewives, especially chubby ones, are always saying they don't eat lunch, but I've seen ½ pound of cheese (900 calories) and 10 crackers (136 calories) "snacked" while they weren't having lunch. What they really mean is that they don't *cook* lunch, and why, then, should we cook? In the first "How to Eat" section I briefly discussed sandwiches. This is so easy, just add your milk and fruit and your effort is over. If you want to have an even easier time, put your fruit on cottage cheese, eat your roll and drink your milk. If that sounds good for every day, fine, but I'm for the greater variety of taste that you can get in a sandwich.

Canned soups are very complicated as far as food exchanges are concerned. Using one-half of the recipe on the can, the easy ones to keep track of have 1 bread and 1 meat exchange. The easiest ones are: cream of asparagus, cream of celery, cream of chicken, chicken gumbo, and minestrone. You can add milk to the first three and then add your milk exchange to that. You can, on most lunch allowances (check your list), have a whole can, but I find if I do this I'm really hungry in a couple of hours, which is again why sandwiches seem to do better.

The recipes here are for when you get tired of sandwiches or for company. If you have to give luncheons, try pushing the girls for potluck lunches, and eat what you can out of what is brought. Otherwise the best recipes are meat or vegetable gelatin dishes. The Knox Company has a wonderful free booklet for diabetics. Send for it. I'm not going to compete with the Einsteins of the gelatin world!

FRUIT SALAD

2 oranges
24 large grapes
1 cup drained artificially sweetened pineapple
    chunks (save the juice)
Juice ½ lemon, strained
2 small bananas
Artificial sweetener as needed

Peel, seed, and cut up the orange segments. Remove as much of the skin on the segments as you can. Cut the grapes in half lengthwise and seed them. Add the drained pineapple. Add the lemon juice and pineapple juice, toss the fruit together, and chill. Just before serving add the bananas, sliced, and taste for sweetness. Add sweetener as needed.

For one:
¼ recipe   2 fruit exchanges   80 calories

Here is an example of a diet lunch you could serve to guests—just don't tell them. Increase the amount of rolls and meat you serve your guests. I assumed the lunch on the 1500-calorie-a-day diet, but with two exceptions (only one roll on 1300 calories per day, and only 1 fruit exchange on 1400 calories per day) it includes all lunches from 1200 to 1700 per day.

2 bread exchanges (warm rolls)   136 calories
2 meat exchanges (sliced turkey)   146
2 fruit exchanges (¼ of above salad)   80
Coffee Jelly (see Index), topped with   —
½ milk exchange   whipped topping
    made from powdered milk   36
                                       ———
                                        398

No fat—save for dinner

HAMBURGER FOR LUNCH

What better? A great big, juicy, runny, sloppy hamburger that you need a bib for, and it's diabetically perfect. If you have a 2 meat exchange, 2 bread exchange lunch allowed (that's most of us), get the best hamburger buns you can find, and buy a pound of the most fat-free meat you can find. Divide the meat into five equal portions. One of these will cook down to a 2 meat exchange. You can either broil the patty or grill it on a hot skillet, but don't overcook it—that makes the meat dry. Toast the bun, do not butter it or fry it (save the fat for dinner). Pile it up with sliced tomatoes, lettuce, sliced onion, Catsup (see Index), or mustard.

It doesn't taste like a diet to me.

> 2 bread exchanges   136 calories
> 2 meat exchanges   146
> ___
> 282

SHRIMP AND TOMATO ASPIC

This recipe is for two for a main dish for lunch or two lunches for you. If you *must* give that luncheon, it will serve four as a salad.

1 cup tomato juice
1 envelope plain gelatin
½ cup Beef Bouillon (see Index)
1 tablespoon lemon juice
1 4½-ounce can tiny shrimp
½ cup chopped celery

Bring the tomato juice to a boil. Sprinkle the gelatin on the cold bouillon and when dissolved mix with the hot juice. Let this cool and add the lemon juice. Drain the shrimp and when the tomato juice mixture starts to jell, add the shrimp and celery. Refrigerate until jelled.

> For one:
> ½ recipe 1 meat exchange   73 calories
> ½ fruit exchange
> (tomato juice)   20
> ___
> 93

SHRIMP SALAD

(*For Two*)

    14 large shrimp ("large" as the supermarket
       defines it)
    1 cup chopped seeded cucumbers
    1 hard-cooked egg, chopped
    ¼ cup Salad Dressing for Meats and Seafood
       (see Index)

If the shrimp are raw, add salt and a slice of lemon to
a saucepan of boiling water. Boil the shrimp about 7
minutes. Chill, remove shell, and devein. Cut them up and
mix with all the rest. Chill a couple of hours before serving, for flavor absorption. Serve on lettuce.

For one:
½ recipe 2 meat exchanges (includes
    egg and dressing)   146 calories
milk exchange (short yourself about
    2 tablespoons elsewhere)   17
                                                   ───
                                                   163
(you have 2 free-fat exchanges left)

CRAB SALAD

Follow the above recipe, using ¾ cup crab.

PERFECT LUNCH SALAD

(*For One*)

Save a breakfast fat for lunch. The best part of this salad is that grated egg tastes so different from bites of hard-boiled egg, and makes the salad so filling—what I call a "stand-up" salad.

⅓ cup torn-up romaine lettuce
⅓ cup torn-up iceberg lettuce
1 tomato, seeded and cut in eighths
Watercress, coarsely chopped as desired
¼ cup julienne-cut beets
2 hard-cooked eggs, coarsely grated
4 teaspoons French Dressing (see Index)

Toss gently together.

½ vegetable B exchange	18 calories
2 meat exchanges	146
2 fat exchanges	90
	254

EGGS MARINARA

(*For One*)

Make a two-egg omelet, following directions for Plain One-Egg Omelet (see Index). Pour ½ cup of hot Marinara Sauce (see Index) over the omelet.

2 meat exchanges	146 calories
½ fat exchange	23
Vegetable A exchange	—
	169

WELSH RABBIT

(*For One*)

Save the extra fat from breakfast.

1 3½×3×¼-inch slice Cheddar cheese, cut up
½ cup hot White Sauce (see Index)
Cayenne pepper or paprika (optional)
Small half English Muffin

Add the cheese to the hot White Sauce and stir until it melts. Add cayenne pepper or paprika if you like. Pour over the warmed muffin.

2 meat exchanges	146 calories
½ milk exchange	85
1½ fat exchanges	68
1 bread exchange	68
	367

CHICKEN SALAD I

(*For Four*)

3 halves cooked chicken breasts, diced
1 cup chopped celery
1 tablespoon minced onion
1 hard-cooked egg, chopped
1 cup Salad Dressing for Meats and Seafood
  (see Index)

Combine all ingredients and chill several hours.

For one:	
3 meat exchanges (including dressing)	219 calories
Vegetable A exchange	—
¼ milk exchange	42
	261

CHICKEN SALAD II

2 small halves cooked chicken breasts, diced
½ cup chopped celery
1 cup drained diet pineapple chunks
20 slivered almonds
½ cup Salad Dressing for Greens (see Index)

Combine all ingredients and chill several hours.

For one:

½ recipe   2 meat exchanges   146 calories
            Vegetable A exchange   —
            1 fat exchange   45
            ¼ milk exchange   42
                                        ———
                                        233

CHICKEN LIVERS AND MUSHROOMS

(For One)

½ cup chicken livers
1 cup cleaned, sliced mushrooms
½ cup Chicken Stock (see Index)
Toast

Crinkle up some foil and put it into a little throwaway aluminum pan. Place the livers on it and heat your broiler.

Simmer the mushrooms in the stock and when they are almost done, broil the chicken livers very close to the broiler, 2 minutes to each side. Put them into the mushroom mixture and simmer 5 to 7 more minutes. Serve on toast.

3 meat exchanges[1]   219 calories
1 vegetable A exchange   —
1 bread exchange   68
                          ———
                          287

[1] If you want a 2 meat exchange lunch, use a scant ⅓ cup of chicken livers, and follow the rest of the recipe.

CHOPPED CHICKEN LIVERS (Fat Free)

For canapes or, even better, just hog it all up for yourself with rye bread for lunch.

½ pound chicken livers
Chicken Bouillon (see Index) to cover
1 hard-cooked egg, finely chopped
1 small onion, finely chopped
Lemon juice to taste
Salt and pepper to taste

Put the chicken livers in a little saucepan, cover with the bouillon, bring to a simmer and cook about 5 minutes. Drain but reserve the bouillon, in case you need extra moistening. Chop the livers fine, or put through the blender at low speed. Mix with all the rest, adding bouillon and seasoning until you get a texture and taste you like. If you are making it for company, pack it firmly in a slant-sided mold and it will come out in a pretty shape for your party. If it's for you, put it in your worst-looking plastic container and hide it at the back of the refrigerator.

For one:
3½ tablespoons   1 meat exchange   73 calories

SHRIMP CREOLE

(*For Two*)

2 cups Marinara Sauce (see Index)
20 large cooked shrimp (or better, 40 medium
    to save money)
Plain Steamed Rice (see Index)

Heat the sauce to boiling, add the shrimp and heat all the way through. Serve with rice, and put the sauce all over the rice.

> For one:
> 2 meat exchanges   146 calories
> (free fat in the sauce)
> Vegetable A exchange   —
> 1 or 2 bread exchanges   68
>   ——
>   214
>
>   or   282

FISH SALAD

(*For Two*)

6 ounces raw halibut steak
Court Bouillon (see Index)
2 small tart apples
2 teaspoons butter
4 tablespoons sour cream

1 tablespoon horseradish
1 teaspoon bottled mustard
1 teaspoon white vinegar

Cook the fish in the bouillon very carefully, until it starts
to flake. Let it cool, and flake the rest of it. Sauté the
apples in the butter, over very low heat, until they are
quite soft. Put them through a strainer, add the rest of
the ingredients, and beat very well. Toss with the fish
and chill. Serve on cold lettuce.

> For one:
> 2 meat exchanges   146 calories
> 1 fruit exchange   40
> 1 fat exchange   45
> (the other fat is free)
>   ___
>   231

CURRIED CRAB

(*For Two*)

1 cup Curry Sauce (see Index)
2 cups loosely packed cooked crab meat

Make the curry sauce and add the crab. Be sure the crab
is at room temperature. Cook over lowest heat until the
crab is warmed through.

> For one:
> 2 meat exchanges   146 calories
> 1½ fat exchanges—free
> Small amount bread exchange   16
>   ___
>   162

CREAMED MUSHROOMS AND CRABS

(*For One*)

1 cup sliced mushrooms
2 cups loosely packed cooked crab meat
1 cup White Sauce (see Index)
Toast

Cook the mushrooms as directed for Everyday Vegetables (see Index). Add the mushrooms with their juice and the crab meat to the white sauce and heat through. Serve on unbuttered toast.

For one:
2 meat exchanges   146 calories
1½ fat exchanges—free
½ milk exchange   85
1 bread exchange   68
                        ———
                        299

(Trim your toast crusts to balance the bread exchange.)
Use two slices of toast if you have the exchange.

SORT OF BORSHT (Beet and Cabbage Soup)

4½ cups Chicken Bouillon (see Index)
1 medium onion, minced
4 cups finely shredded cabbage

1½ cups finely shredded raw beets
Vinegar
Artificial sweetener
Salt
Pepper
½ cup minced fresh parsley (1 tablespoon dried)
Yogurt, if you wish

Bring the bouillon to a boil and add the onion and cabbage. Simmer this 20 minutes; add the beets. Add vinegar a teaspoon at a time with a couple of drops of sweetener at a time until you get a sweet-sour taste you like. Salt and pepper to taste. Simmer 5 minutes. Add the parsley. Drop a dollop of yogurt a tablespoon at a time in each bowl of soup, if you like yogurt. Count your own yogurt.

For one:
¼ recipe   1 vegetable A exchange   — calories
           1 vegetable B exchange   36

Yogurt equals 7½ calories per tablespoon and should be deducted from a fat-free milk exchange.

You can make this soup and use it for several days for yourself, or as a lunch or dinner starter.

WHOLE LUNCH POTATO AND ASPARAGUS SOUP

(*For One*)

Obviously, this is ridiculous to make for one. Any soup this good should be a party treat. I just showed it for one

because the exchanges work out so well for from 1400-
to 1800-calorie-per-day lunches.

½ bunch (8 stalks) fresh asparagus
Salt
1 cup 1-inch cubes diced potatoes
1½ cups Chicken Bouillon (see Index)
2 eggs, beaten with
2 tablespoons light cream
Pepper

Take off the tough ends of the asparagus and cook in a
small amount of salted water until tender. Remove the
asparagus and cook the potatoes in the same liquid until
mashable. Then, mash the asparagus and potatoes together.
Add the bouillon and simmer 1 hour. Pass through a fine
strainer and reheat to boiling. Remove from the heat, add
the eggs and cream and seasoning. Heat without boiling
and keep stirring.

2 meat exchanges	146 calories
2 bread exchanges	136
(potatoes slightly shorted to	
make up for cooked Vegetable B)	
1 fat exchange	45
	327

OYSTER STEW

(*For One*)

Oysters have so many "things" in them that I feel hesitant about bringing them into the book. I like them raw and dipped into Cocktail Sauce (see Index), and I chew them, too. However, Oyster Stew is a lunch dish, and by the "list" you get 5 medium for 1 meat exchange. Save a breakfast fat for this lunch.

2 teaspoons butter
10 medium-size fresh oysters
1 cup milk
1 tablespoon grated onion
Salt and pepper

Melt the butter over very low heat, and cook the oysters in the butter until the edges curl. Add the milk and onion, and heat, but don't let it boil. Serve in a heated bowl. Season to taste.

2 meat exchanges	146 calories
1 milk exchange	170
2 fat exchanges	90
	406
Crackers, 5, a must	68
	474

WHITE CLAM AND POTATO SOUP

Look at the recipe for White Clam Soup. That is soup soup, as before dinner. This recipe is for two and is for a main dish for lunch, as you can see from the exchanges.

2 cups diced (½-inch cubes) raw potatoes
Chicken Bouillon as needed (see Index)
2 cups chopped clams (fresh if possible) with
   their juice
4 teaspoons butter
1 tablespoon arrowroot
2 cups milk
1 tablespoon grated onion
1 tablespoon Worcestershire sauce
Salt

Put the potatoes in a saucepan with enough chicken bouillon to cover. Boil for 5 minutes, then add the clams and their juice and boil for 15 more minutes. If canned clams are used, add them when the potatoes are done, about 20 minutes. Follow the recipe for White Clam Soup for the rest of the recipe.

For one:
  ½ recipe   2 meat exchanges   146 calories
             1 milk exchange   170
             2 fat exchanges—free
             2 bread exchanges   136
                                     ———
                                     452

WHITE CLAM SOUP

Filling, easy, tastes good, and again right off the list.
Also it uses milk easily, so what more could one ask? Free
fat? It's got that too.

    2 cups chopped clams (fresh if possible) with
        their juice
    4 teaspoons butter
    1 tablespoon arrowroot
    2 cups milk
    1 tablespoon grated onion
    1 tablespoon Worcestershire sauce
    Salt

If the clams are raw, boil them for 15 minutes in their
own juice. If canned, just heat to boiling. In another pan,
melt the butter, stir in the arrowroot, and gradually add the
milk, stirring constantly until it simmers. Add the clams
and onion, the Worcestershire and salt to taste. Simmer
3 more minutes. This makes up for four people.

    For one:
    1 meat exchange   73 calories
    ½ milk exchange   85
    1 fat exchange—free
    Arrowroot: part of a bread exchange
        —short yourself elsewhere   8
                                            ———
                                            166

DIARY ENTRY 7

Ho! Ho! Went to the Fair

I have succeeded. I eat without knowing I am on a diet, I am not hungry, and I don't crave sweets.

I never nibbled on a Neapolitan, sampled a soufflé, dunked a doughnut, or drank a diet drink. I kept my resolution, for once, that I could rid myself of the "sweet tooth," by avoiding the big, fat, rich, creamy desserts I loved so much.

And I got vivid proof that I had overcome by backsliding. The Diabetic Association of Southern California had their annual fair—fund raising for diabetic children's camps and other needs—and with it a dietetic bake sale. So I sailed off to eat cake and contribute.

And there were the cakes, beautiful, lovely cakes; all baked in little bonbon cups. Little to keep the exchange count down. I bought three little bonbon spice cakes, about two bites each, and ate them while I was looking at the fair booths. What cakes! I felt all admiring toward the lady who had made such excellent cake without sugar. I finished the six bites, and in a few minutes I was salivating to an embarrassing degree, went back to the cake booth, and recalculated my exchanges. But I had already extended to eat three. I got hungrier, hungrier, nervous, upset—so upset

I flew from the fair. I didn't want six bites of cake—I wanted CAKE—two or three pieces.

I had not been so unhappy about food since my first agonies on the diet.

And I proved to myself that what I had learned from my readings in the physiology of taste was true. I had eliminated my "sweet tooth," but only because I had avoided all of the *very* sweet foods all of the time, or as I said at the beginning of the diary, "cold turkey."

HOW NOT TO EAT DESSERTS
Science, Not Art

What I just told you in my diary is true, and you might be thinking that maybe it worked for me, but you are not me, and we are not the same. None of us is the same as far as our habits are concerned, but eliminating a habit, a "sweet tooth," and the unhappiness that goes with it is the same for every one.

This method of eliminating a habit is scientifically true, and with usual scientific exactness is called "extinction." I no longer eat desserts, and I don't care. As I developed the recipes in this book, I almost forgot that I was on a "diet." I eat better food than I did before, now that I am forced to plan my meals. My weight is stable, I am not hungry, and I don't have food dreams.

Seems impossible? Not in the United States. Every group that immigrated to this country has changed its food habits. Boys from little country towns have come back home after serving in the Orient with a new taste—oriental food. Just as I learned "acquired tastes," I learned to "unacquire" a taste. Reread my diary where I ate two weeks full of very bland foods, and got a new tongue to taste with, and a new "nose" for food.

Another problem is that pie and cake-type desserts are just too expensive in terms of exchanges. A slice of apple pie, made sugar free, uses 1 bread exchange, 2½ fat exchanges, and 2 fruit exchanges, and it isn't very good pie. One piece of sugar-free chiffon cake, no topping, equals 1 bread exchange, 2 fat exchanges, and ½ meat exchange. So what is left for dinner can be put on a small plate.

Simpler foods are just as expensive. One-half cup of orange sherbet equals 2 bread exchanges and you haven't eaten anything. One 3½-inch oatmeal cookie equals 1 bread and there goes that desire for sweets, up, up, up. If you eat ice cream, ½ cup counts as 1 bread exchange *but* you should omit 2 fats.

To start the extinction of your "sweet tooth" eat your fruits for dessert. Fruit Salad (see Index) is a good beginning. You can combine different fruits such as strawberries and bananas (½ cup strawberries and ¼ sliced banana for 1 fruit exchange) and pour a little diet ginger ale over them before you chill them. Another good combination is grapes, pineapple, and melon with orange juice on them.

You can use the basic recipe for gelatin desserts that is on the back of the envelope substituting artificial sweetening for the sugar. Always save the juice from canned diet fruits and use that as part of the liquid. Use diet ginger ale or lemon soda instead of cold water.

If you find it too difficult to start this way, use the desserts[1] in this chapter for your "difficult" day. Use the recipes that concentrate on using milk and fruits. Only none of the recipes uses fat exchanges.

As the "difficult" days diminish, keep your goal in sight. When your yearning for rich sweets is gone, the rest of your life will be even richer.

[1] See Appendix B.

COFFEE JELLY

Once in a while wishes come true, and this dessert is both elegant, easy, and almost free of calories.

1 tablespoon Dutch cocoa
½ cup water
1 envelope unflavored gelatin
1½ cups fresh hot coffee (please, not instant)
1 tablespoon artificial sweetener
Pinch salt
1 teaspoon artificial brandy flavoring

Mix the cocoa and the water and bring to a boil so that the cocoa loses that raw taste. Allow to cool, and add water to bring the water and cocoa back up to ½ cup, if necessary. Sprinkle the gelatin over this to soften.

Add the hot coffee and other ingredients.

Pour into any four pretty glasses, wine, champagne, almost any stemmed glass.

Top with whipped topping made from dry milk and artificial sweetener. Taste. Follow the directions on the package.

For one:
part of a bread exchange   8 calories
part of a milk exchange—
    approximately for most dry milks   28
                                                          —
                                                          36

Short yourself elsewhere for both of these.

EGG CUSTARD

As I mentioned before, this is a good summer breakfast dish if you are lazy, as I am; just eat one-half rather than one-quarter.

2 eggs, slightly beaten
2 cups milk
1 tablespoon artificial sweetener (taste when
  mixed)
½ teaspoon vanilla
Pinch salt

To vary this, add at will:

1 teaspoon brandy flavoring OR
1 tablespoon granted orange rind OR
1 teaspoon almond flavoring OR?

Beat the ingredients together and pour into four large Pyrex baking dishes. Place these in a pan of hot water and cook in a low oven, 300° F., 50 to 60 minutes. Insert a clean knife into the custard, and if it comes out clean the custard is done. Chill.

For one:
½ meat exchange   37 calories
½ milk exchange   85
—————
122

HEAVENLY FRUIT

4 cups either blackberries, raspberries, or strawberries OR
2 cups either bananas, pineapple, or cherries

Cut up the fruit; artificially sweeten to taste. Place in a
strainer and set aside to drain thoroughly.

1 envelope unflavored gelatin
2 cups milk
2 eggs, separated
1 to 2 tablespoons artificial sweetener (taste
when mixed)
Pinch salt
1 teaspoon vanilla

Soften the gelatin in ½ cup of the milk. Beat the remaining milk, egg yolks, sweetener, salt, and vanilla all
together in the top of a double boiler over hot water. Add
the gelatin and milk mixture and rebeat. Bring the water
in the double boiler to a boil and stir until the mixture is
very hot but not boiling. Chill this until it begins to
thicken.

Beat the egg whites until they are thick and stiff and
fold them gently into the thickened mixture.

Take out four tall compote glasses (Pilsner glasses can
come back into use, if you have them) and make alternate
layers of fruit and whip, starting with fruit and ending
with whip. Chill well.

For one:

½ milk exchange   85 calories
½ meat exchange   37
1 fruit exchange   40
                        ———
                        162

Or, you may use a packaged diet pudding to save the ½ milk exchange. Then, for one:

½ milk exchange   85 calories
½ bread exchange   34
1 fruit exchange   40
                        ———
                        159

ORANGE DESSERT

2 envelopes unflavored gelatin
2 cups orange juice
1 tablespoon grated orange rind
1 teaspoon grated lemon rind
2 cups buttermilk
1 tablespoon or more (taste when mixed)
    artificial sweetener
1 cup sliced fresh peaches or drained canned
    diet peaches

Soften the gelatin in ½ cup of the orange juice and slowly warm on low heat until the gelatin is completely dissolved. Add the other ingredients except the peaches and mix together. Chill. When the mixture starts to thicken, add the peaches and chill until set.

For one:

1 fruit exchange	40 calories
½ milk exchange	85
	125

You get 1 free fat to use elsewhere or deduct 45 calories.

JELLIED MELON BALLS

This is a 1 fruit exchange recipe for a dinner dessert. You can double it if you feel like making lots of little balls, or let the kids do it—they think it's fun. Make the balls with the smallest implement you have, so that you do not waste the fruit exchange.

1 envelope plain gelatin
1 cup water
2 tablespoons lemon juice
1 cup diet ginger ale
Artificial sweetener to taste
1 heaping cup watermelon balls
1 7-inch cantaloupe, cut into balls
1 8-inch honeydew melon, cut into balls

Soften the gelatin in part of the water and heat the rest of the water to a boil. Add the lemon juice. Stir until dissolved, and add the ginger ale. Taste to sweeten. Chill until syrupy. Add the fruit and chill.

For one:
¼ recipe 1 fruit exchange   40 calories

CHOCOLATE PUDDING

1 envelope unflavored gelatin
½ cup cold milk
2 tablespoons Dutch cocoa
1½ cups milk
1 to 2 tablespoons artificial sweetener (taste
   before chilling)
Pinch salt
½ teaspoon vanilla

Soften the gelatin in ½ cup of cold milk. Take a little of
the 1½ cups milk and dissolve the cocoa in it. Stir this
into the rest of the 1½ cups of milk and heat until sim-
mering—not boiling. Add this to the cold milk mixture and
stir well. Add the rest of the ingredients and pour into
four dessert dishes.

For one:	
½ milk exchange	85 calories
part 1 bread exchange	15
	100

Short yourself about ¼ bread exchange elsewhere.

TAPIOCA PUDDINGS

I started trying quick-cooking tapioca after my label-reading fit in the supermarket. The advantage of tapioca is that you get long mileage from a small amount of bread calories. Follow the directions on the box, in case they change them, and alter for sweetening. It is no more difficult to make than a packaged pudding and it doesn't have that phony dessert taste. And it's another way to use the milk.

VANILLA NUTMEG TAPIOCA

(*For Six*)

Follow the instructions for quick pudding on the tapioca box. If the recipe calls for ⅓ cup sugar use 1 tablespoon of artificial sweetener. After you take it off the heat, grate in about ¼ teaspoon from a nutmeg nut. The pudding can be served with a fruit topping.

For one:

⅙ meat exchange (1 egg in recipe)	12 calories
Short yourself a couple of bites of meat.	
½ milk exchange	85
½ bread exchange	34
	131

REALLY CHOCOLATE TAPIOCA PUDDING

Follow the directions on the box except substitute 1 tablespoon artificial sweetener for the sugar if it calls for ⅓ cup. Dissolve 5 tablespoons Dutch cocoa in ½ cup of the milk and proceed with the recipe.

For one:

⅙ meat exchange	12 calories
½ milk exchange	85
1 bread exchange	68
	165

RICE PUDDING

2 eggs, beaten
2 cups milk
2 cups cooked Basic Plain Rice (see Index)
1 tablespoon artificial sweetener (taste when mixed)
½ cup raisins
1 teaspoon cinnamon

Beat the eggs with the milk and stir in the rest of the ingredients. Taste for sweetening. Put in a lightly oiled baking dish and bake at 350° F. about 40 minutes or until a clean knife comes out without loose custard on it. Do NOT overcook. It's good either hot or cold.

For one:

1 bread exchange	68 calories
½ meat exchange	37
½ milk exchange	85
1 fruit exchange	40
	230

SUPER-DARK CHOCOLATE MOUSSE

(*For Six*)

This is a little more difficult than Coffee Jelly, but only because toppings made from dry milk have to be made so that they remain very cold while being whipped, and then handled very carefully when being folded in. However, this can be made hours in advance and it is as chocolate-tasting as candy.

½ cup Dutch cocoa
½ cup water
Pinch salt
1½ tablespoons artificial sweetener
1 envelope unflavored gelatin
¼ cup water
Dry milk

Mix the cocoa, ½ cup water, salt, and sweetener and bring to a boil. Sprinkle the gelatin over the ¼ cup of water and let it soften. Mix part of the chocolate mixture with the gelatin mixture, and then mix this into the rest of the chocolate mixture. Stir well and start to chill it. When it begins to thicken:

Make 1 recipe of whipped topping with dry milk from the directions on the box. Be sure to use a large bowl full of ice with the smaller bowl for the mix in it. Fold the topping into the chocolate mixture as rapidly as you can without breaking down the topping. Get it into the coldest part of your refrigerator immediately. Chill until firm.

For one:

⅙ recipe   ¾ bread exchange   51 calories
           part milk exchange   20
                                  ──
                                   71

I think a 71-calorie dessert is worth a little whipping.

APPLE CASSEROLE

Easier than pie, lower in calories, and tastes pie-like.

4 tart apples, peeled, sliced and seeded (Pippins are
   best for this)
¼ cup water
¼ cup lemon juice
1½ tablespoons liquid artificial sweetener
½ tablespoon arrowroot
½ teaspoon cinnamon

½ cup grated Cheddar cheese
1 tablespoon powdered artificial sweetener
¾ cup biscuit mix

Put the apples in a shallow baking dish. Mix the next five ingredients together, making sure the arrowroot is dissolved. Mix the apples with this mixture so that all apples are coated.

Mix the rest of the ingredients and sprinkle over the apples. Bake 30 to 40 minutes at 350° F. or until the apples are tender. Serve hot.

For one:

1 bread exchange	68 calories
1 fruit exchange	40
½ meat exchange	37
½ fat exchange	23
	168

Appendices

Appendix A

DIABETIC FOOD EXCHANGE LIST

DAILY MEAL PLAN

Daily Total (in grams)

Carbohydrate	85	91	116	131	131	136	146	161	167	174	199	207	217	254	260	275	283	290	312
Protein	53	57	59	61	61	70	70	72	76	85	87	95	95	100	111	120	135	150	154
Fat	40	45	45	50	60	65	70	75	80	85	85	90	95	100	115	125	135	150	160
Daily calorie level	900	1000	1100	1200	1300	1400	1500	1600	1700	1800	1900	2000	2100	2300	2500	2700	2900	3100	3300

BREAKFAST

List																			
1 Vegetables	—	—	—	—	—	—	—	—	—	—	—	—	—	—	—	—	—	—	—
2 Breads	1	1	1	1	1	1	2	2	2	2	3	3	3	3	3	3	3½	4	3
3 Meats	1	1	1	1	1	1	1	1	1	2	1	2	2	2	2	2	2	2	2
4 Milk	½	1	1	1	1	1	1	1	1	1	1	1	1	1	1	1	1	1	1
5 Fruits	1	1	1	1	1	1	1	1	1	1	2	2	2	2	2	2	2	.2	2
6 Fats	—	—	—	1	1	1	1	1	1	1	2	2	2	2	3	3	3	3	3

LUNCH

List																				
1 Vegetables	—	—	—	—	—	—	—	—	—	1	1	1	1	1	1	1	1	1	1	1
2 Breads	2	1	1	1	2	1	2	2	2	2	2	2	2	3	3	3	4	4	4	4
3 Meats	2	2	2	2	2	2	2	2	2	2	3	3	3	3	3	3	4	5	4	4
4 Milk	½	½	½	½	½	½	½	½	½	½	½	½	½	½	1	1	1	½	½	½
5 Fruits	2	1	2	2	2	2	2	2	2	1	2	2	2	2	2	2	2	2	2	2
6 Fats	—	—	—	—	—	1	1	2	2	2	1	1	2	3	3	3	3	3	3	3

DINNER

List																			
1 Vegetables	1	—	1	1	1	1	1	1	1	1	1	1	1	1	1	1	1	1	2
2 Breads	—	1	1	1	1	2	2	2	2	2	2½	2½	4	4	4	4	4	4	4
3 Meats	2	2	2	2	2	2	3	3	3	3	3	3	3	4	5	6	6	6	6
4 Milk	½	½	½	½	½	½	½	½	½	1	1	1	1	1	1	1	½	½	½
5 Fruits	1	1	1	1	1	1	1	1	1	1	1	2	2	2	2	2	2	2	2
6 Fats	—	—	—	—	1	1	1	2	2	2	2	2	2	2	3	3	3	4	4

© 1966 THE UPJOHN COMPANY

List 1

VEGETABLES

Group A—You may eat any amount of these vegetables, if they are uncooked, in addition to 1 serving of Group B. But if cooked, only a single cupful is permitted in addition to 1 serving of Group B. If you wish, you may have an additional cupful of Group A in exchange for your Group B serving.

Asparagus	Spinach
*Broccoli	Turnip greens
*Brussels	Lettuce
sprouts	Mushrooms
Cabbage	Okra
Cauliflower	*Parsley
Celery	*Peppers,
*Chicory	green or red
Cucumber	Radishes
Eggplant	Romaine
*Escarole	Rhubarb (without
*Greens	sugar)
Beet greens	Sauerkraut
Chard	String beans,
Collards	young
Dandelion	Squash,
Kale	summer
Mustard	*Tomatoes
Poke	*Watercress

Group B—1 serving equals ½ cup. Carbohydrate, 7 gm.; Protein, 2 gm.; Calories, 36.

Beets	Pumpkin
*Carrots	Rutabagas
Onions	*Squash, winter
Peas, green	Turnips

*These vegetables have a high vitamin A content; at least 1 serving a day should be used.

List 2

BREADS
VEGETABLES
ICE CREAM

Each serving provides:
Carbohydrate, 15 gm.
Protein, 2 gm.
Calories, 68

List 3

MEATS

Each serving provides:
Protein, 7 gm.
Fat, 5 gm.
Calories, 73

Bread, 1 slice
Biscuit, roll, 1
(2" diam.)
Muffin, 1
(2" diam.)
Corn bread,
1½" cube
Flour, 2½ tbsp.
Cereal, cooked,
½ cup
Cereal, dry
(flakes or
puffed), ¾ cup
Rice or grits,
cooked, ½ cup
Spaghetti,
noodles, etc.,
½ cup
Crackers,
graham (2)
Crackers,
oyster, 20
(½ cup)
Crackers,
saltine (5)
Crackers,
soda (3)
Crackers, round,
thin (6 to 8)
Vegetables

Beans (Lima,
navy, etc.),
dry, cooked,
½ cup
Peas (split peas,
etc.), dry,
cooked, ½ cup
Baked beans,
no pork,
¼ cup
Corn, ⅓ cup
Parsnips,
⅔ cup
Potatoes,
sweet, or
yams, ¼ cup
Potatoes,
white, baked
or boiled, 1
(2" diam.)
Potatoes,
white,
mashed,
½ cup
Sponge cake,
plain,
1½" cube
Ice cream (omit
2 fat servings),
½ cup

Meat and
poultry (beef,
lamb, pork,
liver, chicken,
etc.), 1 slice
(3" X 2" X ⅛")
Cold cuts, 1 slice
(4½" sq., ⅛"
thick)
Frankfurter, 1
(8 to 9 per lb.)
Codfish, halibut,
etc., 1 slice
(2" X 2" X 1")
Salmon, tuna,

crab, lobster,
¼ cup
Oysters, shrimp,
clams, 5 med.
Sardines, 3 med.
Cheese, Cheddar,
American,
1 slice (3½" X
1½" X ¼")
Cheese, cottage,
¼ cup
Egg, 1
Peanut butter,
1 tbsp.

Limit peanut butter to 1 serving per day
unless carbohydrate is allowed for in diet
plan.

List 4

MILK

Each serving provides:
Carbohydrate, 12 gm.
Protein, 8 gm.
Fat, 10 gm.
Calories, 170

Milk, whole, 1 cup	¼ cup
Milk, evaporated, ½ cup	*Milk, skim, 1 cup
Milk, powdered,	*Buttermilk, 1 cup

*Add 2 servings from list #6 (Fats) if milk is fat free.

List 5

FRUITS

Each serving provides:
Carbohydrate, 10 gm.
Calories, 40

Apple, 1 small (2" diam.)	*Grapefruit juice, ½ cup
Applesauce, ½ cup	Grape juice, ¼ cup
Apricots, fresh, 2 med.	Grapes, 12
Apricots, dried, 4 halves	Honeydew melon, ⅛ (7" diam.)
Banana, ⅓ cup ½ small	Mango, ½ small
Berries (black-berries, rasp-berries, *strawberries), 1 cup	*Orange, 1 small
	*Orange juice, ½ cup
Blueberries, ⅔ cup	Papaya, ⅓ med.
	Peach, 1 med.
*Cantaloupe, ¼ (6" diam.)	Pear, 1 small
Cherries, 10 large	Pineapple, ½ cup
Dates, 2	Pineapple juice, ⅓ cup
Figs, fresh, 1 large	Plums, 2 med.
	Prunes, dried, 2
Figs, dried, 1 large	Raisins, 2 tbsp.
*Grapefruit, ½ small	*Tangerine, 1 large
	Watermelon, 1 cup

*These fruits are rich sources of vitamin C; 1 serving a day should be used.

List 6

FATS

Each serving provides:
Fat, 5 gm.
Calories, 45

List 7

FOODS THAT NEED NOT BE MEASURED

(insignificant carbo-
hydrate or calories)

Butter or margarine,
1 tsp.

Bacon, crisp,
1 slice

Cream, heavy,
1 tbsp.

Cream, light,
sweet or sour,
2 tbsp.

Cream cheese,
1 tbsp.

French dressing,
1 tbsp.

Mayonnaise,
1 tsp.

Oil or cooking
fat, 1 tsp.

Nuts, 6 small

Olives, 5 small

Avocado, ⅛
(4" diam.)

Coffee

Tea

Clear broth

Bouillon
(fat free)

Lemon

Gelatin
(unsweetened)

Rennet tablets

Cranberries
(unsweetened)

Mustard (dry)

Pickle
(unsweetened)

Saccharin and other
noncaloric
sweeteners

Pepper and
other spices

Vinegar

Seasonings

Low calorie
soft drinks

At each meal you may have as many servings as you wish from this list of foods since these foods contain an insignificant number of calories.

Appendix B

SAMPLE MENUS

AN ORDINARY WEEK

Here are seven menus for a 1500-calorie-a-day diet. It starts with a roast, and has one lunch and one dinner from the roast leftovers. Some menus are for "fat saving" days, others are not. It took me about 1 hour to plan the week, the same amount of time it would take any housewife to plan a week's food. As I do not eat prepared desserts, only fruit, I could have planned it for myself in less time.

The menus are upside down, dinner first, as a complete "real" dinner is the goal of the day. The milk exchanges, if not used in a recipe, are in parentheses. This is so that you can do whatever you work out. Check each recipe that has an asterisk: for instance, the Really Chocolate Tapioca Pudding requires shorting yourself 1 rounded teaspoon of meat.

Consult Index for recipes.

SUNDAY   *Exchange*

All-American Pot Roast   3 meat
Buttered Tiny Noodles   2 bread
                                2 fat
Summer Squash   vegetable A
Carrots Cooked in the Roast Juice   vegetable B
Blackberries   1 fruit
(Milk)

Lunch

Chicken Salad II   2 meat
                                1 fat
                                1 fruit
                                ½ milk
Two Warm Dinner Rolls   2 bread
Sliced Peaches in Diet Ginger Ale   1 fruit

Breakfast

Orange Juice   1 fruit
Sunday Eggs   1 meat
                                1 fat
One Warm Roll   1 bread
(Milk)

MONDAY	Exchange
Chicken Teriyaki	3 meat
Rice in Chicken Bouillon	2 bread
Spinach Sour Cream	1 fat
High "C" Salad (Doubled Salad Dressing)	vegetable A
	3 fat
	1 fruit
Coffee Jelly* (Milk)	

Lunch

Roast Beef Sandwich	2 meat
	2 bread
Fruit Salad (Milk)	2 fruit

Breakfast

Egg Custard	1 meat
Topped with	1 milk
Fruit Jam	1 fruit
Warm Roll	1 bread

Exchange

Grapefruit Cocktail   1 fruit
        Hash   3 meat
                             1 bread
                             ½ vegetable B
    Beau Tomatoes   vegetable A
                             3 fat
Really Chocolate Tapioca Pudding*   1 bread
                             ½ milk

Lunch

    Shrimp Salad*   2 meat
Two Warm Dinner Rolls   2 bread
Bananas and Strawberries   2 fruit
    in Orange Juice
        (Milk)

Breakfast

    Orange Juice   1 fruit
    Jelly Omelet*   1 meat
Buttered Warm Roll   1 bread
                             1 fat

        (Milk)

WEDNESDAY	*Exchange*
Spaghetti	3 meat
	2 bread
	1 vegetable B
Asparagus	1 vegetable A
Herb and Greens Salad	4 fat
(Doubled Plus Dressing)	
Orange Dessert	1 fruit
	½ milk

Lunch

Cottage Cheese and Fruit Salad	2 meat
	2 fruit
Two Warm Rolls	2 bread
(Milk)	

Breakfast

One-fourth Cantaloupe	1 fruit
Egg Nog	1 meat
	1 milk
Warm Roll	1 bread

THURSDAY   *Exchange*

Glazed Pork Chops   3 meat
Basic Plain Rice with Everywhere 2 bread
    Sauce
Artichokes with Butter or   1 vegetable B
    Mayonnaise   2 fat
Cooked Vegetable Salad*   vegetable A
                                 2 fat

Strawberries and Bananas   1 fruit
    (Milk)

Lunch

Hamburger   2 meat
                                 2 bread
One-half Cantaloupe   2 fruit
    (Milk)

Breakfast

Orange Juice   1 fruit
Eggs Arnold   1 meat
                                 1 bread

    (Milk)

FRIDAY	*Exchange*
Grilled Salmon Steak*	3 meat
Baked Hashed Browned Potatoes	2 bread
	(2 fat-free)
Peas (you may butter them)	2 fat
Vastly Improved Cabbage Salad	1 fruit
	1 fat
(Milk)	

Lunch

Chicken Livers and Mushrooms	2 meat
on Toast	1 bread
Sponge Cake with Fruit Jam	1 bread
	1 fruit
(Milk)	

Breakfast

Orange Juice	1 fruit
Broiled Breakfast Burger	1 bread
on Buttered French Bread	1 meat
	1 fat
(Milk)	

SATURDAY   *Exchange*

Stuffed Flank Steak	3 meat
	1 bread
Corn	1 bread
Green Beans	vegetable A
Herb and Greens Salad	4 fat
(Doubled Plus Dressing)	
Jellied Melon Balls	1 fruit
(Milk)	

Lunch

Cream of Chicken Soup (Whole   2 bread
can made with ½ cup milk)   2 meat
                                 ½ milk
Small Banana   2 fruit

Breakfast

Buttermilk Pancakes with Fruit Jam   1 bread
                                       1 fruit
One Egg Omelet   1 meat
(Milk)

Appendix C

As artificial sweeteners vary sometimes from brand to brand, you may have to change the amount of sweetener in any one recipe. The equivalents shown here are the most usual ones on the market.

Artificial Sweetener	Sugar
⅛ teaspoon	1 teaspoon
¼ teaspoon	2 teaspoons
½ teaspoon	4 teaspoons
1 teaspoon	8 teaspoons
1 tablespoon	½ cup
2 tablespoons	1 cup
1 cup	8 cups

INDEX